Care for the Wild

Family First Aid for
Birds and Other Animals

Care for the Wild

Family First Aid for Birds and Other Animals

W.J. JORDAN AND JOHN HUGHES

CARE FOR THE WILD
HORSHAM

First published in 1982 in Great Britain by
Macdonald & Co (Publishers) Ltd

This edition published in 1988
by Care for the Wild, Horsham

Copyright © W. J. Jordan and J. Hughes 1982

Illustrations copyright © Anna Macmiadhachain 1982

ISBN 0 356 08556 2

Printed and bound in Great Britain by
Collins, Glasgow

Contents

Introduction   I

PART ONE: BIRDS

1 Wildfowl (or Waterfowl)   6
2 Other Swimming Birds (including Seabirds)   22
3 Waders (and similar)   31
4 Game(?) Birds   38
5 Birds of Prey (or Raptors)   45
6 Other Birds   56
7 Oil Pollution   70

PART TWO: MAMMALS

8   Small Ones   80
9   Bats   87
10 Hedgehogs   91
11 Hares and Rabbits   99
12 Squirrels   105
13 Stoats, Weasels and similar   111
14 Foxes   116
15 Otters   128
16 Marine Mammals   133
17 Badgers   138
18 Deer   147

PART THREE: OTHER WILDLIFE

19 Snakes and Lizards   156
20 Amphibia   160
21 Fish   163
22 Insects   168
23 Parasites   176

APPENDICES

A Wildlife and the Law   180
B Euthanasia   183
C Close Seasons   185
D Organizations   187
E Wild Animals of Britain   189
   Index   193

Introduction

Wildlife abounds in urban areas, as well as the countryside. Flowers and weeds soon cloak derelict sites. Then insects, birds, and small mammals join them, creating a living harmony; a new cycle of life. The soil teems with creatures that are essential to the survival of all terrestrial life. Worms and a million other organisms break down dead material making vital nutrients available for new plants. Insects provide nutrition for many birds. Every roadside bank, wood, field, and garden is the home for many species which in turn may be food for predators.

At first glance Nature does indeed seem to be a random and cruel business, but look closer. As we discover more, our understading changes for there is a balance in nature – when not upset by Man. As food species become scarce, reproduction falls off, the numbers of living creatures drop, and then the food species is able to increase once again. Prey animals are more difficult to catch so the number of predators fall, too. The balance of nature is finely tuned and works well unless Mankind interferes, as he does in many ways; in making excessive amounts of food available in the form of crops or refuse, or by killing large numbers of wildlife with poisons, traps, and firearms.

But isn't there an enormous amount of suffering caused by one species eating another? Not so. In the wild, through natural selection, prey species have become adapted to being preyed upon so that if they escape, they soon recover and resume their normal behaviour. If they did not, they would become victims of excessive stress, lose weight, and die. If on the other hand, they do not escape, death is merciful because of two factors: shock and substances called endorphines. It is well known that a rabbit caught by a stoat can die in seconds from shock whereas if it is caught in a snare or poisoned it will suffer for a long time. It is known that when normal painful stimuli are inflicted upon vertebrate animals their nervous systems produce pain killing morphine-like substances called endorphines, but this only occurs when the animal is inflicted with pain for which its species has become adapted through natural selection over thousands of years. Unfortunately, Man inflicts injuries on wild creatures – either accidentally or deliberately – to which they are not adapted and they suffer horribly. Accidentally, many are run over by cars, poisoned by waste chemicals, and contaminated by oil; and deliberately, through shooting, trapping, and poisoning.

Much of this death and cruelty results from ignorance. Many people think, wrongly of course, that Nature herself is cruel when in fact suffering is minimized in the natural way of things in the wild. Many think Nature is wasteful because they consider only their own requiremetns for food.

In fact, Nature has produced an enormous variety of species, each fitting in with the others like some giant, exquisite jigsaw. Man is only one piece, but becoming a larger and larger piece (now, nearly 20% of the animal bio mass) and is causing an instability in the whole by creating unnatural imbalances such as monocultures, destruction of rain forests, desertification, and pollution.

Some people think we can do without most of the species of wild creatures. You and I know we cannot. When we walk in the woods and see a wild bird or stroll along the seashore and watch a crab; when we bring flowers or pictures of animals into our homes, we know that our relationship with wildlife is essential to our mental and spiritual well-being. Caring about wildlife engenders a warm, gratifying feeling, giving us a sense of worth not easily gained in other ways.

People often come across sick and injured animals and wonder what will happen to them. Many have an urge to help, but are frustrated by a lack of knowledge, and this is why we have written this book.

Wild creatures are only afraid of Man when he comes within their 'flight line' or 'distance'. A fox or bird will be calm and inquisitive in the presence of Man provided the intruder is outside the flight distance. They may not appear to be suffering, but a bird or animal that allows itself to be picked up by a human is in serious trouble.

It is important to know that wild creatures often disguise their illnesses and can behave apparently normally though their condition is very serious. Therefore, the Good Samaritan should not expect to get more than 20% recoveries, a seemingly sad success rate. However, the joy and sense of achievement resulting from the few successes in caring for injured or sick wildlife makes the effort more than worthwhile.

You may accidentally strike a bird with a car. It drops to the ground, feathers awry, beak open, eyes closed, but it is still breathing. What do you do? Treat it for shock – but how? Take it to an animal hospital – but where? Should it be put to sleep to end its suffering? How do you make that judgment?

The primary intention of giving aid and treatment to an injured, diseased, or abandoned wild creature is to enable it to return, in health, to the wild. The animal must not be treated like a pet because some wild creatures will adapt to humans after their initial fears subside. A lack of fear or a reliance upon feeding by humans, or a tendency in some animals to imprint on or adopt a human, may lead to disaster if they are then returned to their natural wild state. Every possible care must be taken, therefore, to ensure that while caring for wild and injured creatures, a healthy mistrust for human contact is maintained so far as possible by no unnecessary handling or even looking at the patient.

It will be found, not infrequently, that some animals and birds grow accustomed to the one human being who feeds and tends them. With that person, the animal remains quiet and tractable. Should another person, or even the same person in different clothes, approach the animal it may become nervous and even refuse to eat, especially if the animal is being hand fed.

When approaching a wild animal, a useful point to bear in mind is that eyes which look directly forward, as human eyes do, are generally recognized in nature as the mark of a predator, and as such are likely to cause fear and panic. Try to cultivate the habit of not looking directly at an animal. It will not quell the innate fear, but it will certainly lessen it.

One of the major problems in embarking upon the care and treatment of a wild animal is that the vast majority do not take kindly to the caring or the treatment. Attempting to remove a thorn from a lion's paw is more likely to result in having your head bitten off than the eternal loyalty of a grateful animal. Lesson number one, therefore, is never to expect gratitude or even co-operation from your patient. This being so, before attempting to treat the injuries of a wild animal, it is well to know just what injuries you might yourself sustain in the process.

Because animals do not react uniformly, it is necessary to consult the appropriate chapter, but there is one general point which applies to all birds and it cannot be overemphasized. No bird should ever be held near the face. There is considerable danger to the eyes in ignoring this simple rule.

Regarding apparent orphans, do not be in too much of a hurry to take these into your care. Assuming reasonable security from predators, it is far better to leave a healthy young bird or animal where it is found. There is every possibility that the parents will continue to feed the infant and they will make a much better job of it than you are every likely to do. Similarly, the finding of a very young deer all alone is not sufficient reason in itself for carting it off home. It is quite normal behaviour for a mother to leave an infant for a period of time. The rearing of any young, wild creature is very time and patience consuming and fraught with other problems. It should never be lightly undertaken.

We have tried to give advice as to what wild animals should be fed if kept for prolonged periods, as well we have included hints on what they can be fed for shorter periods. After all, you cannot expect to have on hand the correct food for all the species which might come your way, and you can be sure the casualty will arrive just before a weekend or a public holiday when the shops are closed and you cannot get what it needs.

Caring for wild animals can be enormously rewarding, but it can be disappointing too. In many cases long-term accommodation, specialized facilities, and expert skill are required if the survival of the injured animal is to be assured. But this book is about simple first aid to wild animals and what you can do at home, and how you can do it. Its aim is to remove the frustration of not knowing how to care for wild animals, encourage empathy for the creatures with whom we share this unique planet, and above all save the lives of as many animals as possible.

Bill Jordan, March 1988

PART ONE

BIRDS

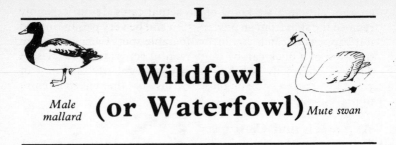

Wildfowl (or Waterfowl)

Male mallard

Mute swan

These birds are quite familiar and easily recognizable to most people as many live in close proximity to human habitation. They include swans, geese and ducks and, apart from the pointed beaks of the goosander and merganser, all have flat or flattish beaks with rounded ends, short legs and webbed feet.

The most widespread of the group are the mute swan and the mallard duck, and there can be few stretches of water anywhere in Britain lacking representatives of one or both of these species. Consequently they are also the most common casualties of the group, and the wild creatures offering the closest rapport for town-dwelling humans.

Possible Handling Hazards

Most people display a distinct lack of enthusiasm about handling a swan. Once the police phoned us to say a swan had landed right in the middle of a busy road junction and would we please come and remove same as it was causing a bit of a traffic problem. On arrival at the scene, we found the swan had decided to set off – walking – down one of the roads which led to the river about a quarter of a mile distant. Crawling along behind at swan's pace was a police car with flashing light, and behind that was a constable, directing the traffic clear of the procession! Here were men who would tackle the largest thugs – but tackle a swan? 'Not likely!' as one of them emphatically stated.

Biting is no real problem with this group. Although some do try to bite, there is no danger from the beak other than a slight bruising on a fleshy part. Geese have a somewhat stronger nip than the others, but this is still nothing to worry unduly about. Swans will seldom even try to bite as though they were aware of their shortcomings in this respect. For the *wings* are this group's principal weapons and these can be wielded to some effect, if not quite to the effect some gory tales would have us believe. It is remotely conceivable that a blow from a swan's wing could break an arm, although we know of no actual cases. It can certainly remove the skin from an unwary shin and be very painful indeed if it happens to catch you in a vulnerable spot. Even a rap from the wing of a duck can be quite painful across the knuckles. A duck will normally only use its wings in defence of a nest or young, whereas a swan or goose will also use them in an attempt to prevent capture.

Approach and Capture

Trying to catch a waterbird on the water is a thankless task leading to frayed tempers and much derision from onlookers. Best try to avoid it if you can unless properly equipped for the job. In general, it will save a great deal of stress and energy (on both sides) if you wait until the bird comes ashore as it must do from time to time, then try to get between bird and water. Chasing must be kept to the absolute minimum necessary, and a bird will almost certainly flee if approached head-on, no matter how slowly you try. The approach should be made walking slowly *sideways*, trying to avoid looking directly at the bird. In this way, it is possible to get close enough to make a final quick move. In the case of a duck, a coat can be thrown over it if no catching net is to hand (a simple catching net can easily be improvised, see Fig. 1). In the case of a swan or goose, the aim

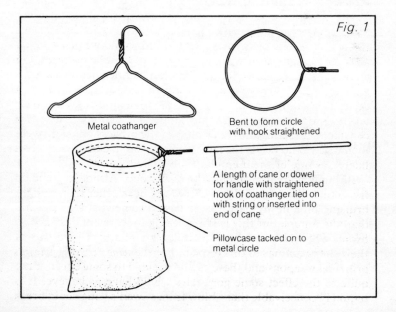

Fig. 1

Metal coathanger

Bent to form circle with hook straightened

A length of cane or dowel for handle with straightened hook of coathanger tied on with string or inserted into end of cane

Pillowcase tacked on to metal circle

must be to secure the wings in their folded position, before they can become weapons.

A swan or goose will very often make a great show of belligerence with much hissing and spread wings, in which case a bold direct approach is needed which will usually cause the bird to turn and run. This is the time to effect a capture and once the bird is secured, with wings folded, there is no further danger except for a not uncommon squirt of faeces which may catch the catcher!

Note: In defence of a nest or young, a swan or goose will almost invariably stand its ground and put up a fight or even launch a unilateral attack, in spite of any injury it may be suffering.

Transportation

A duck can be carried in virtually any container large enough to hold it comfortably so long as air holes are provided. Should the container be required for use afterwards, a generous lining of newspaper or old cloth will guard against the excess of faeces likely to be passed on the journey. The simplest way to transport a goose or swan is in a hessian sack (if you can find one in these plastic days) with one corner removed (see Fig. 2). The bird will readily poke its head and neck through this hole and the open end of the sack can be tied with a piece of string at the bird's tail end. For a short journey, in the absence of a sack, the bird can be 'hobbled' with a piece of thick string or even a handkerchief by bringing the legs over the folded wings and tying them loosely together (see Fig. 3). No matter how quiet it may seem – and most birds will ride quite quietly without moving once a vehicle is in motion – do not attempt to carry the bird loose unless it is screened in some way from the driver or a second person is holding it. A swan attempting to fly is not the ideal passenger in heavy traffic!

Initial Care

Whatever the reason for bringing in the bird, it is desirable to provide a quiet room or pen, if possible warmed to about 20°C (68°F), for at least the first twenty-four hours. Cover the floor with wood shavings or sawdust if you can find any, or thick newspaper if you can't. If using newspaper, it will need changing very frequently – you'll be amazed just how much faeces the average swan will deposit, and even a duck can perform well in this respect. Hay and straw should be avoided as they may contribute to respiratory problems in a debilitated bird. Food and drinking water should be provided from the start for,

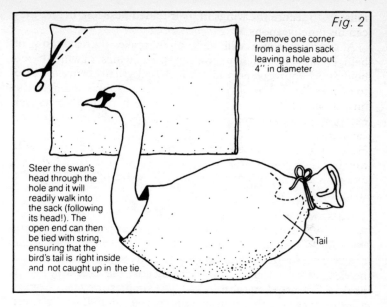

Fig. 2

Remove one corner from a hessian sack leaving a hole about 4" in diameter

Steer the swan's head through the hole and it will readily walk into the sack (following its head!). The open end can then be tied with string, ensuring that the bird's tail is right inside and not caught up in the tie.

Tail

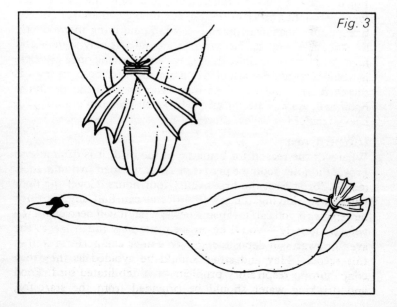

Fig. 3

although waterfowl can go without food for several days, your casualty may already have done so before being found.

Food

Some ducks eat only shellfish, crustaceans and the like and most of the group are partial to the odd insect, etc., though they can fare perfectly well on a vegetarian diet for the period they are in care. Unless you know the preference of your patient, it is best at the outset to provide both types of food since all of them are likely to eat a little fish if offered. Tinned pilchards (in tomato sauce, not oil) will usually be accepted as will chopped-up sprats, herring, cod or other white fish, offered very moist and placed near the main drinking bowl. Tinned meat or fish pet food may appeal to them too.

Grass or cabbage (finely chopped) and cornflakes (soaked in water, *not* milk) will be accepted by swans, geese and most ducks. As with the fish, any food offered should be placed immediately adjacent to the main water bowl as they like to 'dabble' their food (even their best friends could only describe them as very messy eaters!). The grass or cabbage can be floated on the surface of the main water bowl and a little bread added. Most lake and river dwellers recognize bread thrown to them by well-wishers as being edible and it will usually tempt them to start feeding, even in the strangest surroundings. Puppy meal biscuit (softened in warm water) is a good wholesome item to offer if available, and for the longer term, chick pellets (preferably 'starter' or 'grower' size) and/or mixed corn should be obtained from a corn merchant (look in the *Yellow Pages* if you don't know where there is one). If corn is used, it should be well soaked before feeding. We prefer to use pellets because if the bird is not eating well but is drinking, they can be dissolved in the water and the bird can drink the resultant soup. The mixture looks disgusting but is very nourishing. Float a few pieces of bread on the surface to start with.

Force-feeding

It is quite unusual for one of this group to refuse all offers but should this happen and the patient fails to take anything for a two-day period, and there is no obvious obstruction, force-feeding should be attempted pending a possible diagnosis of the trouble. Do not leave it any longer since, as already mentioned, the bird may have eaten nothing for some time prior to capture. Force-feeding is quite a simple operation, the requirements for which are a piece of flexible rubber or plastic tubing roughly the length of the bird's neck, and a syringe. The tubing can be up to about ⅜in. (10mm) outside diameter. A baby cereal, fish purée or a mixture of both should be used, depending on the patient's species which should by this time have been established. If still in doubt, use the fish purée.

It is simplest if there are two of you. One holds the bird in a sitting position with neck extended while the other opens the beak (gentle pressure on the hinge will usually achieve this) and inserts the tube, slightly to one side to avoid the glottis (this is the entrance to the lungs which is situated at the back of the tongue and can easily be seen opening and closing when the beak is open). The tube can be eased gently down the throat, leaving the end protruding for attachment of the syringe (see Figs. 4 and 5). *Be sure to hold onto the end of the tube to ensure the bird doesn't swallow it.* If you don't have and cannot get a suitable syringe, an empty washing-up liquid bottle can be employed, although it is much more difficult to control.

The mixture should be the thickest that will pass through the syringe and the quantity should range from a pint (568ml) per day (divided into three feeds) for a swan, down to a quarter of this amount for a small duck such as a teal. The method of administration is simply to keep filling the syringe, attaching it to the tube and slowly and steadily squirting it down. You won't do the bird any harm providing you don't try to give too much too

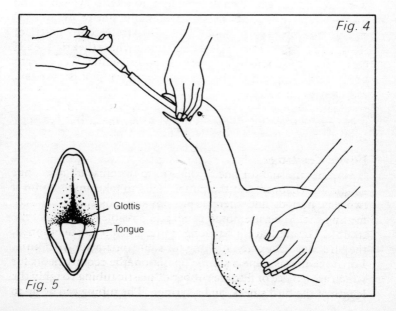

Fig. 4

Glottis

Tongue

Fig. 5

quickly (evidence of this would be some of the mixture coming back up again).

Symptoms, Diagnosis and Treatment

Injuries. The most common injuries are caused by fishing tackle and gunshot. Occasionally a bird may break a wing on an overhead wire. More commonly legs get broken.

Swans seem to be particularly susceptible to injuries caused by fishing tackle. Not only does the line become wrapped around the leg but, not infrequently, the birds ingest the hook with the line attached – perhaps because of the bait. Sometimes weights are also ingested. Many instances have been recorded and one group that was looking for and recording discarded fishing tackle on a village pond and a reservoir of twenty-two acres for a nine-month period, found fifty-two birds and one squirrel entangled with line. Another group over a period of a year dealt with seventy-one birds from thirteen different species.

It is possible that discarded tackle may have become more frequent since the introduction of nylon line, because an ultra fine size was produced that is almost invisible. It is more liable to break when entangled on branches, weeds etc., and is more slowly biodegradable because it is impervious to the effects of water or bacteria. Prior to the use of nylon, silk was used which decayed fairly rapidly.

Treatment consists of catching the bird and carefully removing the line and hook. If the hook has been swallowed an operation may be necessary to remove it and this must be left to a veterinary surgeon. Depending on where it has lodged, it may not cause any symptoms. In this case leave well alone for the hook may become encapsulated (grown round with tissue) or it may disintegrate.

Post-mortem examinations of waterbirds have shown that a considerable number have suffered pellet wounds and recovered. It is unlikely that you will find a bird with superficial pellet wounds unless they are freshly inflicted and the animal is suffering from shock. More usually the bird flies away and either recovers or the wounds suppurate and it dies days or weeks later. Pellets pierce the skin and usually travel some distance from the site of entry and it is often best simply to treat the wound with antiseptic and antibiotic and leave it open to drain. If the pellets are lodged in the wing, however, they may be located by shining a bright torch through the wing from the other side. This shows up the pellet as a dark opaque spot which, as said before, may be some distance from the entry wound. In these cases it may be useful to probe and squeeze until, with the minimum amount of damage to tissue, the pellet can be extracted.

Wounds which are close to legs or wings, where the skin is moving, may allow the entry of air which can travel considerable distances underneath the skin and give it a crackling feel. Try to press this air out gently through the wound, though it is not important to remove it all. Eventually it will be absorbed and disappear as the bird recovers. Large gashes in the skin, especially if near mobile parts, where healing would be difficult due to the continual movement, may be sewn or sutured with a needle and thread that has been sterilized by boiling. Simply pass the needle and thread through the edge of the skin (about $\frac{1}{8}$in. (3–4mm) from the edge) and out through the other flap. Cut the thread and pull both ends gently together until the edges of the skin are touching and then tie securely. Place the individual sutures about $\frac{1}{4}$in. (5mm) or less apart. Always leave an opening at the bottom of the wound so that it will drain. Treatment with antibiotic powder or ointment and bathing with antiseptic solutions is recommended. Birds are more resistant to wound infections than mammals, but nevertheless it is always advisable to take care.

Old open wounds may be treated by bathing them with antiseptic solutions and applying antibiotic powder or ointment if available. The main essential in treating old wounds is to allow adequate drainage and prevent infestation with maggots. This is usually done by the use of antiseptics that contain Phenol or Phenol-type compounds, such as Dettol solution.

A broken wing is fairly obvious, for when the bird is at rest it has an asymmetrical appearance. The wing is not tucked neatly along the body, but droops slightly, perhaps sticking out from the general line of the body. If the bird is chased and it opens its wings the injured one may droop a little or even trail on the ground. On closer examination, when the wing is pulled out, the bird will attempt to withdraw it and part will bend at an abnormal angle. Usually the break is half way along the wing near what we may call the point or 'elbow' of the wing, for this is the most vulnerable part. The best form of treatment is to bind the broken wing in the normal position to the body of the bird using elastoplast strip bandage, leaving the normal wing free. More often than not, although healing occurs within two to three weeks, there is less mobility in the mended bone which may prevent the bird, especially of the larger species, from flying. But usually they survive quite well, though smaller birds may be in a little more danger from predators.

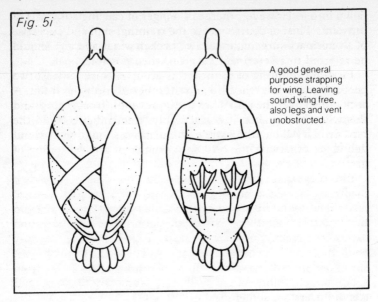

Fig. 5i

A good general purpose strapping for wing. Leaving sound wing free, also legs and vent unobstructed.

A broken joint invariably heals by becoming ankylosed – becoming stiff and immobile, rendering the bird unable to fly.

A broken leg is fairly obvious when the bird leaves the water. It is almost completely crippled, and will try to hop, using its wings for balance. It is a particularly serious injury in large species like swans, and unless healing returns the leg to near normal they will be unlikely to survive in the wild. It is essential, therefore, to have the leg splinted as expertly as possible, and to keep the bird confined until it has healed, which takes three weeks or so.

The break often occurs in the lower part of the leg which, being devoid of flesh, is much easier to splint. But if the skin is lacerated, healing may be slow because of the poor blood supply. When the break is high up in the femur which is surrounded by leg muscles, splinting is very difficult, and the insertion of a steel pin down the shaft of the bone may be possible.

This is done in much the same way as for mammals. The bird is anaesthetized and the skin incised over the break. The muscles are separated so that the break is exposed. A steel pin of the right thickness and length – that is, not too great for the bony cavity – is pushed into the hollow centre of the bone of the longer piece and the shorter piece manoeuvred over the end. If the break is in the centre it may be necessary to push the pin up the shaft and out through the end, then position the lower piece and drive the pin down into it. However, there is a danger of causing ankylosis of the joint. This, of course, needs the training, skill and expertise of a veterinary surgeon, indeed *all* broken wings and legs should be referred to a veterinary surgeon when possible.

First-aid splinting of birds in this group requires at least two people – one to hold the bird and the other to apply the splint. A sock pulled over the bird's head will prevent it from seeing, and this will often quieten it considerably. Remember to hold the bird firmly. All handling and manipulations should be firm and deliberate otherwise the bird will struggle at any relaxation of grasp.

Birds have the capacity to feel pain, but show less reaction than mammals, so it is not usually necessary to give a general anaesthetic – and in any case general anaesthetic can be risky in birds. Local anaesthetic is usually administered by injection around the affected area. Occasionally in birds the injection may be made around the nerve or nerves supplying the wing or limb, thus blocking all sensation to that part. But birds suffer from shock which, more often than not, is caused by fear, and tranquillizers are sometimes used.

To splint a wing simply hold both wings along the body in the normal position and wind elastoplast strip bandage over the broken wing and around the body leaving the normal wing free. To splint a break in the lower part of the leg first place a small amount of gauze and then cotton wool around the limb. Place a splint (a section of split bamboo cut to the correct length to stretch from the joint above the break to the joint below) along the leg and bind in place with elastoplast bandage or insulating tape with the leg held stretched in the normal position. For a break in the fleshy part of the leg, it is essential to refer to a veterinary surgeon.

Once the break has healed, remove the bandage or tape by first cutting it into small portions then carefully peeling off so as not to damage the feathers.

Diseases and Poisoning. Loss of locomotion is fairly common in this group of birds and there are many causes – from shock and poisoning to general weakness caused by chronic disease. When you find a bird that seems unable or unwilling to move or can move only very feebly, first feel its breastbone to see what sort of condition it is in. If the bird is plump and its feathers seem to be in good condition, apart from those that may be damaged, the cause is likely to be of recent origin and may be lead poisoning or poisoning from pesticides or insecticides. If, on the other hand,

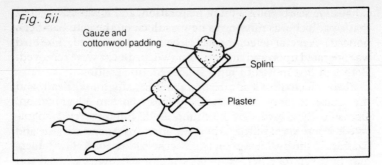

Fig. 5ii

Gauze and cottonwool padding

Splint

Plaster

the bird is thin and emaciated, and looks bedraggled, it is quite possible that the disease is of longer duration and hope of cure, therefore, is more remote.

Post mortems of mute swans in the East Midlands have shown lead poisoning to be a frequent cause of death, and research is now in progress into deaths in other parts of Britain. The main cause is thought to be weights from fishing tackle – lead pellets which are split so that they can be clamped on the line. One mute swan was found to have forty-four pieces in its gizzard. There the pellets are gradually acted upon by digestive juices and lead is continuously absorbed. It is a cumulative poison and as the level in the body rises the bird begins to pass a greenish offensive smelling diarrhoea. It loses weight and many birds develop a neck paralysis before general paralysis. When this stage has been reached treatment is rarely, if ever, successful.

Another source of lead poisoning is the ingestion of lead shot from cartridges. As it has no split in it, it can be easily distinguished from fishing weights. Fallen shot is abundant in areas where wildfowl are hunted, and it has also caused poisoning in mute swans and waterfowl. The lead pellets lie in the mud and seem to be swallowed as an alternative to stones. They lodge in the gizzard and are gradually worn away and some absorbed. This problem of lead poisoning due to ingestion of lead pellets was first noticed in the USA, and many wildfowlers are now using cartridges that contain stainless steel shot rather than lead, so serious had the poisoning become.

I was presented with an interesting case that parallels this problem. An ostrich was suffering from loss of appetite, loss of weight, and was passing greenish, foetid diarrhoea. A clinical examination suggested poisoning – but what? The bird was penned with others that were healthy – but it was possible that a member of the public had given the bird some poison. An exhaustive search plus a bit of inspiration, and it was discovered that a padlock was missing (a new padlock on the gate had been noticed). A metal detector was fetched – and it reacted. The bird was operated upon and not one, but two, padlocks were removed. Both had lost most of their galvanized zinc coating.

Birds affected by lead poisoning are usually found dead, and the cause is only discovered on post-mortem examination. Occasionally a bird may be found alive, but apparently paralyzed. There is very little to be done apart from good nursing and feeding. If the bird has greenish diarrhoea then antibiotic tablets may be given together with a mixture of activated charcoal and either Kaolin or chalk (two parts charcoal to one part chalk). A level teaspoonful given three or four times a day is the dose for a large bird such as swan or goose. Recovery is generally slow because it takes some time for the body of the bird to eliminate the lead from its system.

Botulism is a type of poisoning due to the ingestion of materials containing toxin derived from a bacterium called clostridium botulinum. This flourishes in warm damp conditions, such as lake edges which are drying out, but there is still plenty of damp mud exposed to the warming effects of the sun. The organism grows on rotting vegetation on the borders of the lake under what are called anaerobic conditions (without the presence of oxygen). The toxin is produced and remains viable for a considerable period of time. It is very potent and only a small amount is necessary to kill a bird by respiratory paralysis. Waterbirds come down and feed on the toxic vegetation, and are often found dead in large numbers. A few are found alive, but paralyzed, and may be treated by giving them appreciable quantities of water by tubing (see *Force-feeding*). But there is no really effective antidotal treatment, and there is little or nothing to be seen on post-mortem examination.

Insecticides are widely used in agriculture and horticulture and are highly toxic to other forms of life such as birds and mammals. Fortunately, this group of birds is not often exposed either accidentally or maliciously to this form of poisoning.

Poisoning by excessive feeding of white bread has also been described though it has not been investigated thoroughly. It is said to cause diarrhoea which will clear up when white bread is replaced by normal food.

Salmonellosis, psittacosis, tuberculosis and pseudo-tuberculosis can all occur in this group, but only on rare occasions. These diseases, therefore, will be described in other groups which are more frequently affected later in this book.

Gizzard and intestinal worms not infrequently affect this group and in particular geese. They cause loss of condition in spite of normal appetite. They can be diagnosed by a veterinary surgeon from a sample of droppings and it is quite possible to successfully treat them. However, the general public is not likely to meet with this problem in a recognizable form unless they are nursing a bird for other reasons and find that it is feeding fairly well and yet not putting on weight. When this happens some thought should be given to the possibility of internal parasites.

Bumblefoot is an abscess on the pads of the feet of birds and is occasionally found in this group. Various bacteria are responsible, but most often one called staphylococcus. Treatment consists in opening the hard lump, expressing the pus and treating the inside with iodine solution, and keeping the bird on a hard, dry, clean surface until the wound has totally healed.

Oil Pollution
Wildfowl, as well as seabirds, are frequent victims of oil spillage, as no stretch of water is safe from this hazard. This particular problem is dealt with separately in Chapter 7.

General Care
The plumage of wildfowl is apt to deteriorate if birds are kept indoors for long periods so, providing the treatment will allow it, the patient should be moved outside as soon as possible after the first twenty-four hours, where its plumage can 'weather' in the normal way. It is not necessary to provide a house but a windbreak would be appreciated. If there isn't much rain about, a good spray of clean water from a hose or even a watering can each day will be most beneficial, and if it is possible to provide bathing facilities, again if treatment or dressings will allow, so much the better. A grass paddock is preferable as prolonged confinement to a hard surface is likely to lead to foot sores.

Release
Many birds in this group will fly off on their own when ready to do so. It is, for instance, a complete fallacy that a swan needs a long stretch of water in order to get into the air. A healthy bird can in fact take off and clear a 6 foot (about 2 metres) fence with a dry runway of no more than about 11 yards or 10 metres.

Leaving in this way is a good indication that the bird is ready to fend for itself once again, but since it isn't always practicable to provide conditions conducive to a free take-off, you may have to take your ex-patient to a suitable release point. Since some of this group may lose the sharp edge of their natural wariness during a period of captivity, the release point should be as far away from people as possible and, as some species are territorial (indeed *most* are when nesting or raising a family), it may be judicious to select a stretch of water free of the bird's own species where it can orientate itself without interference.

Orphans

Some ducks are inclined to nest some distance away from water. Why do they do this, you may ask? The banks of rivers and lakes are very busy places by day, with people boating, angling and swimming, or simply walking along with big feet likely to step on eggs, perhaps accompanied by bounding dogs likely to cause aggravation to a broody mum; by night, with the odd fox or stoat on the lookout for an easy meal. One way and another, it isn't such a bad idea to set up house elsewhere. And then, when the ducklings are hatched, the duck will set off to walk to the water, leading the brood. Besides, the practice does produce the occasional heartwarming picture of a London policeman stopping traffic to allow a duck and her family to cross the road!

But, unfortunately, it is by no means an unusual occurrence for the duck to disappear during this hazardous journey, probably into someone's oven, since she makes a very easy catch at this time. Thus the ducklings are left, milling around aimlessly.

Since they feed themselves from birth, ducklings are comparatively easy to care for if a constant source of warmth can be provided where they sleep and a few other simple rules are observed. *In the following, 'ducklings' can also apply to cygnets and goslings.*

An infra-red lamp, which may possibly be borrowed from a farm or kennels, is by far the best form of heating for this purpose but the enclosure must be large enough to permit the ducklings to move away from the heat when they wish to do so. In the absence of such a lamp, some other type of safe heating must be improvised which will keep the temperature at the sleeping place around 35–40°C (95–104°F). Failing anything else, keep the ducklings in the warmest possible room and provide a dry mop head in one corner of the enclosure, which the brood can nestle under and around as a mother-substitute. A broody hen or bantam, should one be available, will offer excellent services as a foster-mother, dispensing with the need for artificial heat.

Although they can be seen swimming quite happily with their mothers in the wild, orphaned ducklings must not be allowed to enter water until they begin to grow feathers, even though they will try their utmost to do so. The down of their early days is simply not waterproof and they will quickly become saturated. Until recent years, it was thought the preen-gland wax of the mother was transferred to the young during brooding each night, thus affording them buoyancy, but we now know that this wax has nothing to do with buoyancy (see Chapter 7). However, there seems no doubt that *some* secretion from the mother is essential in these early days to enable the young to enter the water safely.

Newspapers are not satisfactory as floor covering for ducklings. They are unable to maintain a firm footing, and this can lead to permanent leg distortions. Sawdust is recommended for most of the enclosure, with a patch of floor left clear for the food. Alternatively, old cloth such as towelling can be used if there are no loose threads which can (and will) become entangled around the ducklings' legs. Paper kitchen towels would probably provide a rough enough surface but may prove rather expensive since the floor covering needs to be changed very frequently.

Throughout the period of care, stay away from the ducklings as much as possible so they do not become accustomed to close human presence and do not handle them any more than absolutely necessary.

Although they cannot be allowed to get into water, the ducklings must be provided with a generous and constant supply for drinking, and the best piece of equipment to provide this is a chick drinking fountain, obtainable from most pet shops or agricultural merchants. If necessary, a fountain can be improvised using a jam-jar and saucer (see Fig. 6).

For food provide all, or as many as possible, of the following each day: finely chopped hard-boiled egg, finely chopped grass, chick mash/insectivorous mixture. It is difficult to give a precise guide to quantities, but suffice it to say they will eat a great deal

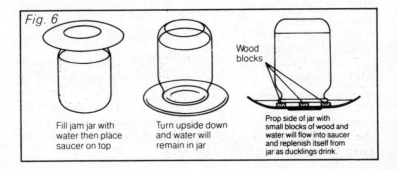

Fig. 6

Fill jam jar with water then place saucer on top.

Turn upside down and water will remain in jar

Wood blocks

Prop side of jar with small blocks of wood and water will flow into saucer and replenish itself from jar as ducklings drink.

more than you might imagine, so be generous. They will not overeat.

Chick mash can be obtained from a corn merchant or possibly a pet shop. Small ducklings find mash easier to assimilate than even the smallest pellets, although pellets can be used for cygnets and goslings from the start. Ducklings can move onto starter pellets after about two weeks. Insectivorous mixture (e.g. *Sluis Universal*) can be obtained from any pet shop or in bulk from a specialist merchant such as John Haith of Cleethorpes. Mix the pellets and insectivorous mixture together in equal proportions and serve dry but, as with all food, adjacent to the drinking fountain. The chopped egg and grass will keep the ducklings going until you are able to get the other items. It is best to simply scatter the food on the floor, clearing away each morning any left over from the previous day. Do not leave stale food around.

If you do not know the species of your ducklings, it would be as well to provide some fish as mentioned earlier for an adult. Place this in a container low enough for the ducklings to reach into but small enough to preclude their getting in for a bathe. The pots in which some sandwich spreads are sold are ideal.

The length of time the heater will be needed will depend on the ambient temperature and the species involved. The best way is to let them decide for themselves. If you pay a quiet visit after they have settled down for the night on two or three occasions, and find they have moved their sleeping position well away from the lamp, it is safe to dispense with its use. After about a week without a heater and providing the weather is mild, the ducklings can be transferred to an outside pen with a shelter they can get under in heavy rain (they will, in fact, usually do this). Light showers will do no harm at this stage and will help get rid of the dirt they accumulate because they are denied bathing.

The species in this group do not all get their feathers at the same age, so keep a lookout for feathers appearing. When the breast is covered, the ducklings can be allowed to bathe *ad lib*. It is not necessary to wait until they are fully fledged (when they have their main wing feathers).

The time for release is when they *are* fully fledged and, as with adult casualties, it is better they make their own decision and fly off when ready. If they must be taken for release, follow the same suggestions as for adult casualty releases and, if possible, provide some of the food they have become accustomed to somewhere in the vicinity for the first few days, even though it is likely to be eaten by every other bird in the area!

Other Swimming Birds (including Seabirds)

This chapter covers a pretty wide field but the physical details common to most in the group are pointed beaks and webbed (or partially webbed) feet. The size ranges from the gannet at 3 foot (just under 1 metre) and with a wing-span of 6 foot (2 metres) to (say) the little tern at about 10in. (25cm). Neck length varies from very long to hardly any.

The most common in the group, and the most widely encountered, is the herring gull, vast numbers of which now never go near the sea, spending their lives on rubbish tips where the pickings are much richer. At the other extreme, many of the group such as the auks (guillemots, razorbills, etc.) never come anywhere near humans unless some disaster befalls them, such as being covered with oil.

Possible Handling Hazards

All of this group can, and will, bite and most can draw blood. The severity of the bite, of course, varies enormously. The long powerful beak of the gannet, with an edge serrated like a hacksaw blade, can cause quite a severe laceration to a bare arm, while the much smaller and more delicate kittiwake will give only a minor nip. But do not take the size of the bird as the criterion for the severity of the bite – the efforts of some of the smaller members of the group can be quite memorable!

Although not used as weapons, it should be remembered that birds with webbed feet still have claws at the end of them, and these can scratch quite painfully if the bird is handled clumsily. Be prepared, too, for strong vocal protests from the bird.

Approach and Capture

The circumstances in which one of this group might be found in distress are so wide and varied that it is virtually impossible to generalize on approach and capture. The flight distance or line varies quite considerably and is also affected by the incapacitating factor. In other words, a fit bird might feel quite safe at x feet but the same bird, if injured, may feel it needs a much greater margin in order to effect an escape and so may well start running (assuming injury to wing and not leg) before you have even spotted him. Others may opt for trying to hide, and this offers the easiest capturing prospect since most of the group aren't very good at it.

As with the previous group, any waterbird feels safer on the water and so will, of course, try to reach this safety when approached. It is imperative the catcher imposes himself between water and bird if he is to have any chance of an effective capture and having done so, a slow, sideways approach, as in Chapter 1, is recommended. Some of the group such as the grebes are not very good on their feet whereas gulls, for example, can run very rapidly indeed. It is preferable to enlist the aid of several people to catch a bird rather than one person driving it to exhaustion.

For those unaccustomed to handling, or if you do not recognize the bird and are unaware of its capacity for doing you a bit of no good when you try to get hold of it, the simple 'throw a coat over it' routine is the best option for initial capture unless you are equipped with a catching net (Fig. 1). When this has been effected, remove the coat slowly and grasp the bird firmly with one hand just behind the head. With the other hand, or the knees if it is a large species, secure the wings from flapping. With an elastic band, a piece of string or, if nothing else is available, the hem torn from a handkerchief or some other piece of cloth, secure the beak taking care not to cover the nostrils (some species in this group have no apparent nostrils but can still breathe with beak secured).

Do not make the error of feeling completely safe with the beak 'taped' as many of this group can and undoubtedly will stab with the point. So it can do no harm to reiterate the warning – *do not hold any bird near the face.*

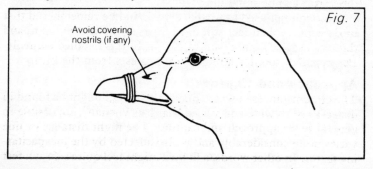

Avoid covering
nostrils (if any)

Fig. 7

Transportation

Any well ventilated container can be used for transport providing it is large enough for the particular bird, i.e. the bird should be able to sit in a natural posture with no distortion of the plumage.

The 'tape' on the beak should be removed for the journey as some birds in this group tend to vomit after being under stress (the chase and capture by a human, for instance). If this vomiting is not observed and the tape quickly removed, there is a great danger of asphyxiation.

As with waterfowl, if the container is required for subsequent service, line it with newspaper or cloth for the journey otherwise it will be fit only for the dustbin when you reach your destination.

We have had birds transported to us successfully in all manner of containers: shopping-bags, duffle-bags, even paper carrier-bags. But do not make the same mistake as a well-meaning gentleman who travelled sixty miles to bring in a guillemot he had found on the beach. He had placed it in a draw-string container like a sponge-bag but instead of drawing up the string leaving the head protruding, he had enclosed the whole bird and it had suffocated, probably only a short time after he set off on his long journey.

Initial Care

Just as with a human, if a bird is not naturally exposed to infection, it has no opportunity to build up immunity. Seabirds in particular are highly susceptible to an infection of the lung called aspergillosis, so do not house your patient in an old dusty building where the lethal spores might lurk. Hay and straw are also very suspect, and should be avoided in any building housing seabirds. Thick newspaper is best for the floor and there is no need to provide any kind of 'bed' as the bird will simply sleep at any point within the enclosure and not necessarily the same place twice. A period of warmth (about 20°C, 68°F), peace and quiet will be most beneficial initially, with food and drink at hand.

Food

All of this group eat fish and some will eat nothing else. This can range from whitebait to mackerel or herring, depending on the size of the patient. The fish should be offered whole, if the appropriate size can be readily obtained, as some birds do not appear to recognize strips of fish as being fish. You do not, after all, find many strips of fish swimming about in the sea.

There is no greater connoisseur of fresh fish than a seabird so it is useless offering anything which is a little 'off', but frozen fish (after thawing of course) will be found acceptable in most cases.

The fish should be offered in a shallow dish with just a little water, sufficient to keep it moist. There is no necessity to offer any other water, salted or otherwise (see *Symptoms, Diagnosis and Treatment*).

Some of the gulls, the herring gull in particular, will accept tinned dog or cat food readily. Indeed a herring gull will eat virtually anything edible, hence the great success of the species, but if the patient is being fed on anything dryer than fish, it is recommended that a bowl of additional water be available. It is not necessary to add salt.

Failing anything else, tinned pilchards (in tomato sauce, not oil) will find favour with most gulls and grebes but are unlikely to tempt the ocean birds such as the auks.

If in doubt as to which fish to buy, go for the smallest. A larger bird can eat small fish but not the other way round and whitebait or small sprats will be found acceptable to most of the group. Some of the larger species such as cormorants and shags will appreciate dead day-old chicks. (see Chapter 5).

Force-feeding

If this should prove necessary, and give the patient at least twenty-four hours before considering it so, the job is best tackled by two people – in the case of a gannet, three if they are available!

For most of the group, small firm sprats are best to use for the purpose since they are easiest to administer. For a gannet, small to medium mackerel are best.

One person can catch up and hold the bird while the other does the actual force-feeding. The holder can wear gloves but the feeder cannot, since it is virtually impossible to open the beaks of most of this group wearing gloves. So it is up to the holder to save the feeder from being bitten by holding the bird firmly with one hand just behind the head until the feeder has grasped the beak, and the fish should be given head first.

As should be apparent by now, the beaks of most of this group are quite strong with powerful jaw muscles, consequently many of them are difficult to open. Conversely, once they *are* open, they are comparatively easy to retain so while the fish is popped in and pushed well down the throat (see Fig. 8).

It is difficult to know just how many fish to give when force-feeding, and it is equally difficult to lay down set rules, so much depends on the species of bird being dealt with and the size of the fish. As a general rule, two fish – of a size the bird can comfortably swallow – twice a day should be sufficient to keep the patient

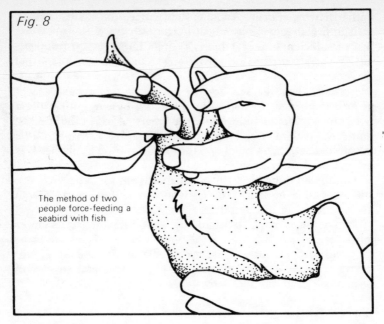

Fig. 8

The method of two people force-feeding a seabird with fish

going and, of course, further fish should always be left within reach. These should always be counted so that it can quickly be seen if the patient has taken any voluntarily. Immediately it does so, force-feeding should cease.

Symptoms, Diagnosis and Treatment

Injuries. These are rare in purely sea birds or, at least, do not come to the attention of the public, mainly because they spend all of their time at sea or along the coast. However, the herring gull and the black-headed gull do come inland to follow the plough in search of worms, to scavenge on rubbish tips, and to nest in towns along the sea front. They quite often suffer injured wings from flying into wires or other objects and, of course, they are shot at by the public from time to time and suffer wounds from pellets. It is rare to find a gull with a broken leg.

Treatment of broken wings follows the same pattern as for the previous group (see pages 13–15). Two people are necessary and the wing must be held in place while it is bound to the body. Healing is rarely successful, however, because these birds spend so much time in the air – using their wings for gliding as well as flying – and the union of the broken bones has got to be exactly right for the bird to be able to fly. It is for this reason that, although many gulls have had broken wings successfully treated, it is impossible to release them back to the wild, and many are kept for their lifetimes, which are quite long (can be as long as thirty years), in captivity. It is during these long periods that infections such as aspergillosis of the lungs and staphylococcus, infection of the legs, occur.

Poisoning, apart from intentional poisoning with Alpha-Chlorolose, is rare. The birds do not feed in areas where botulism poisoning can occur, nor do they pick up lead shot or lead pellets.

Alpha-Chlorolose is a narcotic poison that kills the bird by rendering it unconscious or semi-conscious and susceptible to death by loss of body temperature. It is for this reason that it is most often used in winter, because the birds die quickly from exposure. The use of the drug to control bird pest species such as gulls and pigeons and a few others is licensed by the Ministry of Agriculture, Fisheries and Food. It is illegal to use it indiscriminately.

To kill herring gulls, bait impregnated with the drug is spread around the roof tops and around rubbish dumps where the bird has become a pest. All the sites of bait are marked so that when the operation is completed any uneaten bait can be collected and destroyed. When the birds eat sufficient of the drug they become narcotized and unable to fly. Some birds lie quietly asleep while others flap and stagger about in a 'drunk' manner. The birds are semi-conscious and not suffering, in the true sense of that word. Nevertheless it is upsetting to the public, and for this reason the authorities who lay the bait generally have sufficient men available to pick up and humanely destroy narcotized birds as quickly as possible.

Should non-target birds become affected it is possible to treat them, provided they have not eaten too large a dose, by keeping them warm and giving them fluids when they are alert enough to take them. Provided that the dose is not a lethal one, the bird will gradually recover.

Oil Pollution

This is by far the most major hazard for seabirds, requiring separate discussion (see Chapter 7).

General Care

A seabird can be kept away from water (for swimming) for quite some time with no apparent deterioration of the plumage, certainly for the three or four weeks an injury may take to heal. So it isn't strictly necessary to provide a pond (see Chapter 7) although most will enjoy a dip if it can be offered.

When moved out of doors (always desirable as soon as possible with any patient), a grass paddock or aviary is preferable for the larger members of the group and also for the grebes, while a smooth concrete surface is recommended for the auks and gulls.

Release

This should be at the earliest possible moment since some of the group very easily become 'tame' to the point of following a human around like a dog, a condition which will be unlikely to benefit their health when released since some vandal will undoubtedly feel obliged to kill such a bird.

The average gull will fly off when ready to do so from anywhere, but others of the group simply cannot orientate themselves when out of sight of the sea and will make no attempt to fly, even from an open pen. Gannets, auks and divers should be taken to the seashore, preferably at some quiet spot, for release; grebes to any large stretch of water. If the bird is fit, it will normally take to the water or the air immediately, although a gannet will occasionally stand motionless on the shore for quite some time, thinking about it, before departure.

Orphans

Apart from gulls, and the herring gull in particular, nestlings of this group seldom, if ever, are likely to be found in circumstances suggesting they might be orphans. The reason for this is simply that most prefer to nest well away from human habitation, many on quite inaccessible cliff ledges, and should the nest be left unattended for any length of time, the occupants will themselves quickly make a meal for a predator. But very occasionally fledglings may be picked up, and they can be cared for in the same manner as an adult bird since they are likely to be quite self-sufficient so far as feeding is concerned.

Because many gulls have taken to nesting on buildings, it is by no means unusual for very young chicks to be picked up for various reasons – such as falling down a chimney. Perhaps we have just been fortunate but the gull chicks we have had have accepted food readily, without resort to elaborate subterfuge. Tinned pilchards in tomato sauce mixed with breadcrumbs generally go down very well, and quite often tinned dog meat is happily eaten. The food should be quite wet at first but with plenty of decent sized lumps the youngster can easily get hold of. A dish of water should be left next to the food bowl and most chicks will dabble their beaks in this.

The subterfuge mentioned above is based on natural feeding behaviour in the nest. Adult gulls have a red spot on the underside of their beaks which the chick will tap and worry at, thereby stimulating the parent to regurgitate the food. An artificial beak is presented to the chick, complete with red spot for the chick to tap, and it is an established fact that the chick will instinctively do this, no matter how inexpertly the beak has been fashioned. A quantity of food is then deposited for the chick to gobble up.

We have no doubt that this does probably work, and would recommend it be tried should you be presented with a reluctant chick. But, as mentioned above, we have experienced no such problem, as most gull chicks of our acquaintance have eaten us out of house and home with absolutely no artificial stimulation!

A human-reared gull chick may hang around the garden for a considerable time but will usually depart eventually. Some will set off to make their own way in the world as soon as they are fully fledged. It is always best to let them make up their own minds, if you have the room to do so, rather than taking them away somewhere strange for release. If they leave under their own steam, they will be able to find their way back should they find the pickings lean elsewhere.

A friend who runs a bird hospital offered a bit of interesting information about the fulmar which is a bird very much like a gull in appearance but with tubular nostrils. It seems that in the latter stages of fledging when the youngster very much resembles the adult in appearance but cannot yet fly, it is fattened up by the parents then left on the breeding ledge to complete its feather growth. At this time it is apt to be set upon by gulls and forced off the ledge. It will then plane down to the water and float in to the beach. It seems they do not feed during this period so should you happen to come across one, there is no point in trying to feed it. It will live on its own fat until fully fledged, by which time the wings will protrude beyond the tail, and can then be released. If you should be attempting to keep more than one, they should be kept separately, otherwise they will squirt an oily fluid at one another and make an awful mess!

It should be mentioned that there are some casualties which aren't really casualties at all. Some birds simply cannot take off from flat ground, the manx shearwater being a case in point, and from time to time one is blown inland during a gale and is found apparently unable to fly. I remember one occasion when a car arrived with a party of young men and a shearwater they'd found some thirty miles away. The spokesman was most solicitous. 'It seems to be injured,' he said. 'It was just sort of crawling around on the ground.' Although it was quite apparent (to us) what the problem was, the bird was given a thorough examination (the least we could do after they'd come so far), after which it was pronounced fit and thrown into the air much to the alarm of the anxious onlookers. Their faces were a picture as the bird disappeared into the distance, heading for the coast.

Little tern

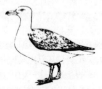

Herring gull

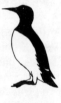

Guillemot

Gannet

Waders
(and similar)

We have added the 'and similar' since some of the birds in this group are not, strictly speaking, waders. We have, for example, included coots and moorhens, not only because of similar physical appearance, but because they can also be cared for in a similar way.

The notable feature of the group is long legs with unwebbed feet. Beaks range from short and straight to long and straight and long and curved. All are pointed – with the exception of the spoonbill which is an occasional visitor with a very distinctive beak as its name implies. Neck length too varies from very short to very long which always reminds us of a certain woman who rang to tell us of an injured bird she had encountered, describing it as 'a duck with a long neck'. The bird turned out to be a bittern!

As with the previous group, there is quite a range of sizes with the heron at one end measuring around 3 feet (just under 1 metre) to the tiny ringed plover at the other, measuring a mere 8in. (20cm). From a casualty point of view, the heron is probably the most common, very often coming to grief in collisions with overhead cables. It also suffers badly during hard winters.

Possible Handling Hazards
The greatest danger from this group, particularly the larger of them, is to underestimate the reach of the neck. The bird will frequently make a stab for the handler's eyes if given the opportunity, and the heron, for example, has a very long reach indeed. All of the group have this distinctive stabbing action of the beak which is after all their method of catching food, but which can be disconcerting, to say the least, when one is on the receiving end. However, most of the smaller ones have no defence at all other than to try desperately to escape.

Approach and Capture
Many of this group have a propensity for paddling in boggy, marshy ground which often means the rescuer must flounder

about in wellington boots in order to catch a still mobile, injured bird. Others inhabit more solid beaches but can get up a very respectable turn of speed with long legs moving so rapidly they can hardly be seen, and since most if not all of the group are exceptionally shy and nervous, an approach can be most difficult. Others will simply hide when a human appears, and their camouflage is quite impeccable.

We can offer no easy formula for capture except, as suggested in the previous chapter, try to enlist the aid of several people. It will cause less stress to the bird in the long run if it can be secured quickly.

It is particularly important with this group to keep the bird well away from the face and never underestimate the reach. The larger birds should be held with one hand just behind the head but do be careful not to twist the neck in any way. As a general rule, the bird will remain quite still once it finds itself securely held, but don't be lulled into relaxing the hold behind the head or you may quite easily lose the sight of an eye. As mentioned earlier, most of the smaller members of this group will attempt no defence at all when captured but will be very distressed indeed at the close proximity to a human. This can be alleviated by removing yourself from the bird's view and the simplest way of doing this is to place a handkerchief over the bird's head until it is placed in the travelling container.

Transportation

It is desirable, indeed essential in the case of long journeys, that the bird should have enough room to stand up since long-legged birds, particularly the larger ones, can very easily get cramp and even paralysis if the legs are kept artificially folded for any length of time. With the smaller members of the group, this is no great problem since they aren't very tall, but containers of sufficient depth to hold a heron don't come easily to hand. The simplest solution is to tie a handkerchief over the bird's head, leaving the beak free and let it travel loose. It is unlikely to move if it cannot see, but if for any reason this course is not practicable or indeed, if the bird has a broken leg, then it is best to secure the wings to the body, as well as covering the head, and lie the bird on its side with the legs stretched out.

The type of container for the small members of this group can be virtually anything of sufficient size to contain the bird in question. Even a paper bag with a few air holes will usually be sufficient to contain a small wader. It will prefer the security of being in hiding rather than make any attempt to escape from the container.

Initial Care

Being offered somewhere to hide will contribute immeasurably to the recovery of any casualty in this group. What this consists of is quite immaterial, just so long as the bird can get out of sight: a screen of any sort, even a small table or stool laid on its side, anything which allows the bird to disappear from view when you approach the room or pen in which it is being housed.

Sawdust is the best floor covering for this group, or cloth if this is not available. Newspaper *can* be used but some of the group find it too smooth for comfortable walking.

As with all casualties, a period of adjustment in warmth and quiet with food and water available, is essential. It is best not to attempt any treatment, unless this should be imperative – to staunch a flow of blood, for instance – until the day after arrival when the bird will hopefully be in a better state to cope with the additional stress involved. But the patient will almost certainly benefit from the immediate administration of some fluid before being left to rest (see *Symptoms, Diagnosis and Treatment*).

Food

Fish is the best thing to offer any of this group – mashed white fish or whole sprats depending on the size of the patient (and the size of the fish). Also, for the smaller patients, the more solid types of tinned dog meat chopped up and minced or small strips of raw meat. The large members of the group such as the heron or bittern will usually accept sprats and sometimes a dead chick or mouse if one or other is available, but do not give a mouse you just happen to find dead since it may have been poisoned.

Small crustacea such as shrimps will be eaten by some, principally the shore dwellers, and chopped hard-boiled egg may also be accepted by many of the smaller members of the group. Do not be afraid to try *anything* if you think it may stimulate the appetite. If your patient will accept it voluntarily, it is unlikely to cause any harm for a limited period. Failing anything else, we would suspect that many members of this group would accept caviare, if you can afford to try it! Offer fish in a dish or bowl of water, and the other food moist (apart from the chicks, mice and egg), and keep a bowl of clean water in the pen.

A certain amount of experimentation may also be required into *how* the food is presented. Your patient may accept food from a blue dish when it flatly refused the same item from a red one. It may scorn any dish but gobble up the food readily when it is simply scattered on the floor. It may refuse all blandishments when inside a building only to eat like a horse when transferred to an outside pen.

Do not stand around waiting to see the bird eat as it almost certainly won't while you are there. Take a careful note of the quantity of anything you give so you are able to ascertain later if any has been consumed. It is always better to offer a choice of several things rather than trying them out one at a time. The bird may be dead by the time an acceptable diet is found.

Force-feeding

In general, we do not recommend attempting to force-feed members of this group. For one thing, with the smaller long-beaked species, there is considerable danger of damage to the beak when attempting to open it and hold it open, but another much more significant reason is the extreme nervousness of this particular group, which usually causes them to vomit anything they have been forced to eat immediately afterwards. There seems little point in subjecting the patient to such a traumatic experience if little or no benefit is derived but, on the other hand, it is very difficult to simply watch your patient die. So if you feel you simply must try it as a last resort, use the tube feeding method recommended in Chapter 1, varying the length and diameter of the tube depending on the species, and using a fish and/or meat purée. Take the utmost care with the beak of a long-beaked species. Do not attempt to open it or hold it open by the tip, but insert the thumb nail between the mandibles near the hinge and prize them gently apart. Hold the beak open by inserting something across the mandibles of the smaller species (a pencil, for example). The mandibles of a heron can be held open as there is much less danger of damage. Administer the food slowly and as soon as the operation is completed, retire from the scene quickly.

If the bird retains the food, then a repetition of the operation is justified but if it is vomited, the kindest thing is to destroy the bird rather than cause it any further distress.

Symptoms, Diagnosis and Treatment

Injuries. The most common bird in this group to be found injured and requiring help is the heron. The most common injury is to the wing in spite of the fact that the legs look long, fragile and easily injured. Treatment of broken wings is the same as for the water-birds in Chapter 1.

A useful splint to apply to the very occasional broken leg is a piece of light hose pipe of the correct length split down the side so that it may be folded over the shaft that is broken. It's useful to pad the limb with a little gauze before taping the hose pipe in place. Healing occurs in about three weeks or so.

Herons do not 'winter' very well. In a severe winter many may be found dead, or suffering from general debility. The best treatment for those still alive is to bring them into warm and dry surroundings and coax them to feed. Often they will perk up fairly rapidly, but while the bad weather lasts they should be kept indoors and nursed back into full health and vigour.

Injury to shore waders is seldom seen simply because they do not come inland, and when injured will often fly out to sea to rest. They sometimes suffer from eating contaminated molluscs and may be found debilitated or dead. Treatment consists of giving activated charcoal to try and absorb the poisonous substances. However, the percentage of success is very small indeed.

Oil Pollution

We have not encountered any of this group suffering from actual oil pollution itself, although, as just mentioned, shore waders can be affected by eating molluscs which have ingested the solvents used to disperse an oil slick.

General Care

Provided they are feeding and have a hiding place to which they can retire at will, keeping a member of this group indoors for a few weeks (three should be ample for most injuries to heal) does no apparent harm. It is always best, though, to get any wild creature out of doors – which is after all its natural element – as soon as possible.

As mentioned in the food section, you may find that a patient from this group will only feed when out of doors, in the quietest possible spot with no people peering at him, and plenty of cover.

A grass paddock or aviary is obviously best, with plenty of clumps of long grass, shrubs or even weeds and nettles (see Chapter 22). A shallow sunken pool will lend a touch of familiarity for some of the genuine waders. We have had many a convalescent heron stand for hours staring into such a pool although there isn't a fish in sight!

Release

We always feel happiest if a bird will take off from where it has spent its convalescence. This gives a good indication that it feels itself ready to face the world, but such a course isn't always practicable or desirable. It is also a good idea to try and return a bird of this group to where it was found, or at least to that vicinity. A measure of common sense must be employed, though, because the bird might have been found in an environment completely foreign to its species. If the finding location isn't known or appears completely unsuitable, consult a good bird book on the type of habitat frequented by the particular species you have been treating and seek out such a spot.

Where the convalescent pen *does* make a suitable take-off location, and this is the course you decide to adopt, do not be too surprised if your ex-patient hangs around for a long time, showing a marked reluctance to fend for itself. We had one particular heron which spent its convalescence in our waterfowl paddock where it completely ignored the other residents and spent all its time staring into the pond, as described earlier, showing no inclination to set off into the great wide world although its broken wing was now perfectly sound. This went on for about a month with the only activity of the day being a rapid retreat into hiding when one of us approached with a bowl of sprats, followed by an equally rapid reappearance to stuff its beak as soon as we left.

We caught the bird up quite often during that month to re-examine the wing. Perhaps it hadn't mended as well as we'd thought, and wouldn't support the bird. But all was well, and we heaved a collective sigh of relief when eventually it took off. The following day, however, a visitor asked, 'What's that great big bird sitting in a tree over there?' Sure enough, there was our heron, perched incongruously in a tree only a short distance (as the heron flies) from the waterfowl paddock, and staring down in that inimitible heron manner. We tried to ignore it but the accusing stare finally wore us down and we placed a bowl of sprats in the usual spot, whereupon it promptly flew down, devoured the fish, and returned to the tree.

It was a further three weeks before our scrounger finally decided to go and work for itself!

Orphans

Owing to their secretive nature, orphans of this group will seldom be found, the exception being coots and moorhens. We have reared these in the same manner and on the same food as ducklings (see Chapter 1). Indeed, on more than one occasion, an odd moorhen chick has been reared *with* a brood of mallard ducklings. A place to hide must be provided, however, for although the chick will potter about quite happily with the ducklings when no-one is around, it will still instinctively run and hide at your approach.

Most of the members of this group are what is called 'precocial' or 'nidifugous', meaning a bird which leaves the nest immediately or soon after hatching and follows the parent. This being the case, there is a greater chance of survival if an orphaned infant be allowed to join a group of other precocial infants, albeit of a different species. Indeed many infants of the group are of a very similar appearance and difficult to tell apart without the presence of an adult bird.

Food as for ducklings should prove acceptable to all with the possible addition of finely minced beef.

The young of the larger members of the group, such as the heron, would require hand-feeding. We have never actually encountered such a nestling but would suggest smallish eels as a suitable rearing diet together with the odd dead chick or small rodent which may have to be chopped up. Although we have fed a good many adult herons on sprats with no apparent ill-effects, we would have some reservations in recommending them for rearing a youngster, the sprat being essentially a salt-water fish. There may be no significance in this but possibly fresh-water fish might be more advisable, even if more difficult to obtain.

There is little risk of imprinting with any of this group, particularly if they are reared with other youngsters. Release can be carried out as for adults when the youngster is fully fledged.

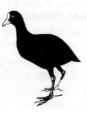

Coot

Plover (Lapwing)

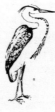

Heron

4

Game(?) Birds

The question mark in the heading of this chapter is neither an accident nor a printer's error, but is quite intentional. The rearing of animals for food forms no part of this book, even though we do hold strong views on certain aspects of it. So-called game-birds come within our terms of reference, so a preliminary comment is not misplaced.

Even though they do wind up as food (albeit not for the average table) we find the practice of rearing any sentient creature with the sole intention of blazing away at it with guns in an orgy of slaughter *purely for fun and diversion*, to be quite abhorrent. And there are other considerations. How, for instance, can you explain to simple French or Spanish peasants, indiscriminately shooting birds in migration, that what *they* are doing is any different from what these presumed more enlightened gunmen are doing? Also, many gamekeepers are quite uncompromising with any other species which might carry off an egg or chick, and some of their methods of killing and maiming are quite diabolical. We have seen many a raptor with one or even both feet severed as a result of being caught in a pole trap (see Chapter 5). If a badger should eat a pheasant egg thereby killing the occupant, the badger itself is likely to be killed for so doing, whereas if the badger *hadn't* eaten the egg, the occupant would be killed anyway, not very much later, by a gentleman with a shotgun. It does not seem quite equitable.

To return to the general characteristics of the group, most people will recognize the pheasant, at least in full plumage, with its long elegant tail, while the other members of the group are markedly similar to domestic poultry of varying sizes. The pheasant and the capercaillie are about the same length, if you count the pheasant's tail which is about 18in. (45cm), but the capercaillie is much larger in terms of weight. It could easily be mistaken for a turkey if you hadn't seen one before. The smallest member of the group is the quail at a mere 7in. ($17\frac{1}{2}$cm).

Possible Handling Hazards

The capercaillie can be very aggressive during the nesting season but since it is confined to woodlands in less accessible parts of Scotland, the chances of encountering one, particularly an injured one which needs to be caught, are quite remote. The rest of the group are very nervous indeed (and who can blame them), so approaching one that is still mobile can be very difficult. It is best, as always, for several people to help capture the bird as quickly as possible. Some kind of netting – nylon or string fruit netting or fishing net, even a tennis net for the larger species – is invaluable. Pegged out on posts or draped on a hedge, the bird won't recognize it as a barrier and will run straight into it if herded in the right direction. Birds with leg injuries are a fairly simple proposition since they find it almost impossible to get into the air with a damaged leg and cannot take advantage of their rapid ground speed.

When captured, this group do not normally attempt to bite although they will sometimes offer a rather ineffectual peck or two. A pheasant will sometimes attempt to scratch with its feet in the manner of a cockerel but it isn't very good at it. Indeed most of this group's efforts are concentrated on trying to escape rather than putting up a defence. It is necessary to hold the wings quite firmly against the bird's body as they are quite powerful and move so rapidly that the bird may do itself damage in its frantic efforts to escape. Unlike other groups which will more or less submit and stay quiet once they are under restraint, this group will renew their efforts to escape at the slightest loosening of the hold, and will continue to make the effort throughout their period of captivity, no matter how severe the injury.

Transportation

Some will sit quietly in a darkened box for a time, but more often they will thrash about trying to get out. A box which offers close confinement is therefore preferable to one with plenty of room. A soft bag such as a zip-top shopping or sports bag is quite good, particularly for a pheasant in full plumage. In any other type of container, the long tail can present something of a problem but in this type of bag, the zip can be left open at the end and the tail left protruding. It is best to wrap the bird (apart from its head) in a piece of cloth or a towel before placing it in the bag, otherwise it will not be content with a position of reasonable comfort but will try to turn around the other way, getting itself tied up in awful contortions in the process.

Initial Care

The truly wild members of this group will *not* passively accept a captive state. They will expend great amounts of energy they perhaps can ill-afford, probing for an escape route. Indeed their efforts in this respect would warm the heart of any prisoner of war escapee. If mobile, they will spend hours simply pacing up and down, peering at the wall in the hope that an opening may suddenly appear, and there is really no way to alleviate this restlessness. It will be more pronounced, though, when there is a human in sight, so leave the bird alone as much as possible and try to avoid sudden appearances which will startle your patient into blind panic, crashing around and doing itself further injury.

There is no ideal accommodation for a truly wild member of this group. A warm room offering the least possible sight of people is the best which can be offered in the early stages. Cover the floor with newspaper, and offer food and water.

Food

This should, fortunately, present no problem. The group will eat virtually anything fed to domestic poultry – chick pellets, mixed corn, chopped greens, chickweed, grass, breadcrumbs – and they will usually accept food quite readily between escape attempts!

They generally prefer to eat off the ground so if you serve the food in a dish, they are likely to stand in the dish and scratch everything out onto the floor so you may as well just dump it on the floor in the first place. A bowl of water for drinking should also be provided.

In the unlikely event of your patient failing to eat, offer some chopped hard-boiled egg to tempt the appetite. A bit of tinned dog meat will also generally prove acceptable, as will any of the proprietary insectivorous foods.

Force-feeding

Force-feeding is not recommended for a member of this group. It should never be necessary and if your patient should fail to eat at all, there is something radically wrong – damage to the beak, for instance.

Symptoms, Diagnosis and Treatment

Injuries. Predictably, the principal injuries suffered by this group are gunshot wounds which are almost invariably fatal. Occasionally one may see a bedraggled pheasant with dishevelled feathers and a drooping wing. It is very difficult to catch such a bird as it tends to run through undergrowth which is often impassable to human beings. But should an injured bird be caught, the first thing to decide is whether the injuries are so extensive that it should be humanely killed. If this is not the case then the wing should be treated and splinted in the way described in Chapter 1. Broken legs may also be splinted if the break is below the fleshy part of the leg. If it is in the fleshy part splinting may well allow the leg to heal, but often the joint becomes fixed and the bird is unable to use it. Wounds should be dressed in the way described previously (see pages 13–15), and they tend to heal rapidly.

Pheasants will occasionally fly low across a road and be hit by a car. If the bird is alive it will probably be suffering from shock. The muscles will be twitching and its eyes will be closed or part closed. If its neck is not broken and the injuries are not too extensive, a quiet hour or so in a box will generally be sufficient to allow it to recover. If after twelve hours it has not recovered consciousness, then it would be better to put it to sleep humanely.

Diseases. Pheasants are susceptible to salmonellosis, psittacosis and myco-bacterial diseases, and on post-mortem examination they are often found to have been suffering from one or other of these diseases. However, this does not mean to say the pheasant is more susceptible than other wild species. It may well be a result of a captive breeding, for these diseases are also common in pigeons and ducks.

Salmonella is a septicaemic type disease (basically, blood poisoning) and clinical symptoms and indeed the lesions or injuries are not usually sufficiently characteristic to establish a diagnosis. Usually the animal is found dead, but a bird that is showing signs of debility may well be suffering from a chronic type of salmonella.

Psittacosis is a virus disease affecting the lungs and air sacs of many wild birds and, of course, the parrot family with which it was first associated. It occurs in two forms: the acute, in which the bird is rarely seen alive; and the chronic, which affects a large number of wild birds of many species, and has no recognizable symptoms. However, under conditions of stress, birds may develop the acute infection and they rapidly become weak, dull, lose their appetite, lose weight rapidly and develop diarrhoea and a nasal discharge. In most cases, death occurs rapidly, probably before a diagnosis has been made. Little can be done in the way of treatment for this disease and it is better to put the bird to sleep humanely.

Myco-bacterial infection or avian tuberculosis also affects pheasants, wood pigeons, starlings and sparrows. In other words, all the birds that are associated with man. Primary lesions of tuberculosis are usually in the intestinal tract and this may lead to diarrhoea. In any case the birds become debilitated with loss of weight and lethargy. There is no treatment for this disease and when diagnosed the bird should be humanely destroyed. Pheasants are also affected by gape worm – a worm that lives in the windpipe causing the bird to develop breathing difficulties and gaping (breathing with the mouth open). This is treatable with the newer worm remedies such as Tetramisole, Dichlorxylenol and Gapex.

Red grouse are often affected by tiny white thread-like worms in their caeca (part of their intestines). Some scientists believe that this infection coupled with shortage of food causes many deaths and certainly loss of condition. Yet others say that some grouse in good condition have as many worms and don't seem to be troubled. It is probable that the worms only cause disease and death when the population of grouse is high – there would be greater contamination of the ground and food may be in short supply. The worm, called trichostrongylus tenuis, is susceptible to some of the newer worm treatments such as Mebenvet which can be given by mouth.

General Care

The problems of housing a member of this group, particularly the larger members, do not mellow with time. In fact the problems during convalescence are even more difficult. When fit, these birds are apt to take off vertically, thereby thumping their heads on whatever is overhead and they will keep on doing this over and over again until you yourself get a headache just watching them. They will continue to do it when you *aren't* watching them, so it is obviously essential that whatever is overhead is as high as possible, with an absolute minimum of 7 feet, preferably 8 (2–2½ metres).

Placed in an aviary, the bird will continue its pacing up and down routine but this should do no harm as this group do not usually cause damage to themselves by probing their beaks *through* the wire as some others do.

As mentioned in initial care, there is no *ideal* accommodation for a member of this group. Even tame and domesticated specimens kept in an aviary are apt to try the vertical take-off if startled and they will do the same indoors. The only thing to do is offer accommodation with as much headroom as possible, and release the bird as soon as you can.

Release

This should preferably be during the close season for the particular species (see end of chapter) as you won't be very pleased to have your patient shot immediately on release – and the bird won't be too enthusiastic about it either!

It is preferable to take the bird to an area best suited for its species, where it will fend for itself quite easily on release. Most bird books will give an indication of suitable habitat and areas of distribution. If you don't have, or cannot refer to such a book, the area where the bird was found is likely to be satisfactory.

Orphans

It is by no means unusual for a chick of this group to become detached from the rest of the family. It may then be found wandering aimlessly, and will almost certainly fall victim to a predator if not rescued. If what appears to be a whole family is found, do not be in too much of a hurry to gather them up as the mother may be in the vicinity. Sometimes the mother's travels take her over a country lane and she may come out of a gate on one side, with the youngsters following, to be confronted by a hedge with no gate on the opposite side. If there isn't a large enough space in the hedge for her to squeeze through, she may fly over and wait on the field side while the youngsters struggle through small gaps in the hedge to join her. Should a car come along during this crossing, the motorist may be confronted by a group of milling chicks, apparently with no parent.

The chicks of this group feed themselves from birth and are therefore easy to cater for although an odd one on its own may prove a problem in that it may continue to look for its lost family, rather than feed. For this reason, it is preferable if the odd youngster can be reared with other chicks, though not necessarily of the same species, and a broody hen will make an excellent foster-mother. If no foster-mother is available, provide exactly the same accommodation and conditions as for waterfowl youngsters (see Chapter 1).

Chopped hard-boiled egg, chopped grass and/or chickweed, chick starter pellets and an insectivorous food obtainable from any pet shop, will make an excellent diet. Budgie seed is also acceptable.

Do not be in too much of a hurry to put the youngsters outside. Wait until they have a good covering of feathers rather than the down of infancy, otherwise a cold snap or a heavy shower may carry them off. A portable chicken run (see Fig. 9) is satisfactory

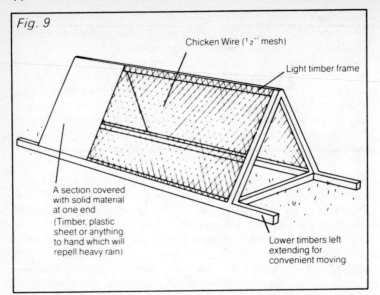

Fig. 9

Chicken Wire ($\frac{1}{2}$″ mesh)

Light timber frame

A section covered
with solid material
at one end
(Timber, plastic
sheet or anything
to hand which will
repel heavy rain)

Lower timbers left
extending for
convenient moving

when the chicks move outside but they should not be considered ready for release until fully fledged, when they can be taken to a suitable site (see *Release*).

There are charts detailing dates of the open and close seasons for game birds (and mammals) on page 185.

Quail

*Male
partridge*

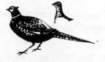

*Male
pheasant*

5

Birds of Prey
(or Raptors)

Most people will recognize a member of this group although others are sometimes mistaken for members. The cuckoo, for instance, is quite like the sparrowhawk and we often have adult swifts brought to us as 'baby hawks'.

The distinctive features common to all of the group are the hooked beak, strong talons and binocular vision (eyes which look to the front and focus together). The size of the group ranges from the golden eagle (which you are unlikely to encounter and will be fortunate even to see) to the merlin, plus of course the owls which are easily recognized by most people even though the vast majority seldom see one alive.

A great deal of interest and enthusiasm is generated by this group, probably much more than all the others put together, and the reasons are not easy to define. Falconry of course accounts for much of the interest and there can be no denying the thrill of having such a bird return to land on your hand after flying high, wide and free. But there are many, many more people fascinated by a raptor than those engaged in falconry, and fascinated is *not* too strong a term. Could it be the binocular vision, which gives them eyes not unlike our own?

Owls, particularly, seem to intrigue most people, possibly due to childhood stories of the 'wise old owl', but some people aren't too enthusiastic about meeting them face to face at close quarters. Among the many we have dealt with over the years, were two tawny owls which spent some time with us, perching all day on a tree branch we had fixed for them in a corner of the office up near the high ceiling (we were very short of aviary space at the time). Most of the day they would sleep but occasionally they would open their eyes when someone came in and give a few clicks of their beaks, advising the intruders to keep their distance.

On one occasion, a dear old lady came in to transact some business or other and she happened to glance up and see this tree branch with the pair of owls perched thereupon.

'Oh, what a beautiful display,' she said, admiringly.

Four round eyes suddenly opened wide to stare at her and two beaks clicked a warning in unison.

'Good heavens, they're alive!' cried the dear old lady as she fled.

Possible Handling Hazards

It is most unusual for a bird in this group to bite although they will hold their beaks open in a threatening fashion, as though intending to do so, all the time they are being handled. It is the feet which pose the danger. They will defend themselves with their claws, or talons, and will hang on with a vice-like grip, often necessitating a second person being called upon to release the grip.

Depending on the size of the bird involved, damage from the talons can range from a row of small punctures in the skin, to a wound requiring several stitches. A grip from the smallest can be painful even if it doesn't do any real damage. There is also a marginally greater danger of a bite from one of the smaller species but this is more likely with a tame or semi-tame bird than with a true wild one. Owls will occasionally bite but not often. The greatest danger from an owl, notably the tawny, is in defence of a nest of young when it can be quite formidable and inflict severe injuries, usually with the talons, on anyone it considers a threat.

Approach and Capture

When first approached, an injured raptor will usually try to hide even if the chosen place of concealment isn't really adequate. The 'head in the sand' principle seems to apply. None of the group, except perhaps the little owl, are very fast on their feet so in the face of a rapid approach and no (even inadequate) concealment, many will simply crouch down and 'play dead'. Some will retain this rigid posture – with beak agape – even when picked up, but this cannot be relied on so the best course is to cover the bird's head with a handkerchief.

A head covering (also covering the eyes, of course) is the only restraint necessary for all of this group, but it is not always quite so easy to achieve. When confronted, the bird is apt to turn over on to its back to fend off the assault with its talons, and trying to drop a handkerchief over the head under these circumstances is rather futile since the bird will keep on kicking it away. The safest method is to have the container to be used handy, then offer the bird a stout stick to grasp. When it has done so, lift it into the container upside down (the container needs to be large enough for the bird to be able to right itself). When the lid is partially closed, cutting off the bird's view of the handler, it will usually release its grip on the stick, allowing it to be withdrawn and the lid fully closed.

Should the bird refuse to grasp the stick – as it may well do – the simplest plan is to cover it completely with a coat or something similar, and slowly ease this back until the talons are revealed and a firm grasp can be taken of the legs. The bird will lie quiet so long as its head is covered and once the talons have been neutralized, the coat can be withdrawn, another hand can be placed under the bird and it can be lifted (slowly and gently) into the container. Try to prevent the bird grasping one talon with the other during this process as it can do itself virtually as much damage as it can do to you and this can cause additional problems later (see *Symptoms, Diagnosis and Treatment*).

Transportation

A ventilated cardboard box is all that is needed, even for a large raptor, since the passenger will show no interest in attacking the container. In the absence of a suitable container, the hand-kerchief simply draped over the head or with two of the points tied together under the beak, will be sufficient to keep the bird immobile for as long as necessary. This is precisely the purpose of the ornamental hood worn by birds used in falconry. It should be noted, however, that hooding is inappropriate and indeed unnecessary for owls. An injured owl, placed quite loose in a vehicle, will simply scuttle into a corner or under a seat and is unlikely to cause any problem on the journey.

A cautionary note. Wicker cat baskets are not recommended for the transportation of large raptors or indeed any large bird. They usually have very sharp protrusions which do not seem to bother a cat but can cause quite severe lacerations to a bird.

Initial Care

If the bird has travelled in a box of some sort, you could not do better than leave it in there overnight in a warm room, unless there should be some urgent reason to do otherwise. It will benefit from the lack of further disturbance at this time, and a move to more comfortable accommodation can easily be post-poned until the following day. Obviously the box must allow for a reasonable amount of movement including the bird standing up.

Suitable quarters for a bird of prey are not easy to provide, as they can cause themselves damage if the accommodation is wrong. For the time being, until the patient has recovered from whatever brought it to you in the first place, quite restricted quarters will suffice – such as a large wooden box which will allow the bird to stand upright on a perch and stretch its wings. The perch should be of sufficient thickness to preclude the points of the talons touching the ball of the foot where they can cause injury and lead to further problems (see *Symptoms, Diagnosis and Treatment*). The ends of the box should be covered with paper or cloth to be changed regularly and the same on the base. The reason for the end coverings is that for most of this group, the term 'droppings' is not quite appropriate since they are in the habit of leaning forward and shooting out a jet of faeces to the rear! The top of the box, from where all servicing can be done, should be covered only with a piece of small mesh nylon netting.

This may seem a sterile, featureless place to keep a bird and of course it is, but the less stimulation to movement the better while an injury is healing and this group are prone to stand for long periods without movement, even when quite free to move.

Food

A great deal has been written about the care of raptors in captivity, including many ideas as to what they should have to eat. Our quite unequivocal view is that the best possible food you can offer to a member of this group is dead day-old chicks with no additives. No bone meal, no vitamin supplements, no extras at all. We have had dealings with most of the group at one time or another and have dealings with some of them regularly, and in quite large numbers, and all have been fed on this diet with no problems whatsoever. Some, we might add, for periods of years.

Unfortunately, because dead day-old chicks are such good food, the casual raptor keeper is likely to experience great difficulty in getting hold of any since most are snapped up from hatcheries by falconers, bird gardens, zoos, etc., in which case you will have to fall back on raw meat with artificially added roughage (fur or feathers). If you can't find anything else, give your dog or cat a brush and use this! A raw meat diet alone is *not* good but it will do no harm to an adult bird for a short period.

At one time, reasonably cheap raw meat could be obtained from pet shops but the practice seems to have ceased. You may therefore have to buy a piece of beef unless you are prepared to scour the roads for bird accident victims, which will meet ready acceptance from most raptors but is a rather unsavoury pastime, calling for much dedication! Any meat offered must be in pieces, not minced, although don't hesitate to offer minced meat if nothing else is available.

There is little point in offering a raptor anything other than raw meat, in one form or another, but there is one small consolation. A raptor can go without food for several days with no ill-effects so you don't have to break your neck to get something on the first day. Having said that, though, do not leave it too long because the bird may already have been without food for a day or two before it was found.

Raptors do not normally drink but do enjoy a bathe, so if the quarters and any dressings will permit, provide a shallow dish of sufficient size for your patient to have a splash about.

Force-feeding

Possibly we have been lucky but we have never ever been obliged to force-feed an adult raptor. Some have gone without food for two or three days but they have all taken food voluntarily in the end. In view of this experience, it is difficult to suggest circumstances in which we would recommend the practice or consider is essential or even advisable. But one of the early lessons one should learn is that no matter how much you know about wildlife, you don't know everything and are never likely to.

Should force-feeding be contemplated, as always it is best to have two people – one to hold the bird with wings firmly to sides, and the other to feed. The talons should be pressed onto a thick wad of cloth or a cushion to prevent their taking part in the proceedings. In spite of its formidable appearance, it is not really difficult to open the beak and, providing you don't force the mandibles too far apart, there is little danger of causing damage. Blunt forceps are best to use for holding the pieces of food and for the inexperienced, blunt the tips still further by wrapping a piece of sticky plaster around each. Place the piece of meat well back on the tongue to start with (later pieces may not need to be so far back once the bird realizes what is happening), close the beak and gently stroke the throat to ensure it is swallowed. You should be able to observe the swallowing action.

Ensure that the pieces of meat, chick, or whatever you are using, are quite moist by dipping them in water before offering them. It is very difficult to give a firm guide as to quantity but using day-old chicks as a measure, a kestrel which is feeding itself will thrive on a 1 and 2 regime with one fast day. That is to say one chick on one day and two the next, alternating for six days, and nothing at all on the seventh. A buzzard should have twice this amount (a 2 and 4 regime). One chick per day for a little owl, and two per day for a tawny, again with a fast day. Others in the group can be gauged from these examples.

Symptoms, Diagnosis and Treatment

Injuries. Birds of prey, in spite of their relative rarity, are quite often brought for treatment. Perhaps their greatest hazard is persecution by gamekeepers by shooting and pole trapping (a spring trap on top of an upright). In attempting to protect their pheasants, gamekeepers look upon birds of prey as deadly enemies, and many will do all they can to destroy them. In spite of the fact that it is illegal, pole trapping is still around and we have seen cases of both feet being severed by such a trap. The birds, of course, had to be destroyed.

They are also protected from shooting, but they are still shot, and injured birds are often brought in for treatment. The injuries inflicted are the same as those in other groups as indeed are the treatments (see pages 13–15). The principal casualties are the buzzard, kestrel, tawny owl and little owl which are more numerous than other species of raptors. They respond well to captivity, but any broken wing, however, must be perfect when healed, or as near perfect as possible if the bird is to survive, for it depends entirely on its excellent flight and sight to catch its prey. If the bird is not 100 per cent fit and is unable to fly well it must either be kept in captivity for the rest of its life or humanely destroyed. It would be cruel to turn this bird loose in the wild and let it starve to death.

Diseases and Poisoning. Some gamekeepers and farmers get rid of birds of prey they think are taking some of their pheasant chicks by poisoning. It is cruel, unnecessary and illegal. The Royal Society for the Protection of Birds has produced a booklet called *Silent Death* which exposes this problem. Though death from pesticide poisoning is not instantaneous, it is rare to find poisoned birds alive. It is also possible for birds of prey to be affected by taking small mammals that have been poisoned by pesticides. Some poisons accumulate in the body of the bird of prey until there is sufficient to kill it.

General Care

As mentioned previously, good accommodation for a raptor is not easy to provide, particularly in the convalescent stages, because all of them, when startled, will tend to fly at the wire in an attempt to escape. Owls do reasonably well in the ordinary average aviary. The smaller diurnal raptors *can* be kept in such an aviary, but even they are apt to damage the primary wing feathers and the tail feathers, as well as the cere (the fleshy part of the beak near the face). Larger birds can do serious damage to themselves in such a place.

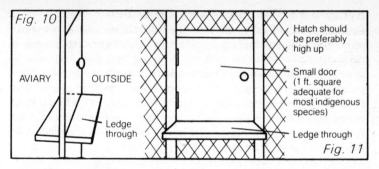

If an existing aviary is to be used, vertical bars of dowel or cane should be added inside the wire about 2in. (5mm) in from it and about the same distance apart. If the top is of wire, this should be covered in the same way. There must be somewhere for the bird to hide so if there is no natural cover (long grass, weeds, foliage), a wooden box with an open end will suffice. Access to one end of the aviary should be denied to people and the box placed with the opening facing this end as for the fox enclosure (see Fig. 14 on page 123).

If an aviary is to be purpose built, it should be a long rectangle with two of the long sides and one of the short (or even all four) covered in a *solid* material. Translucent fibreglass or PVC sheeting is ideal but lapboard timber can be used. The height should be a minimum of 7 feet (2 metres) and the top should be of a heavy gauge, small mesh nylon netting with a covered section of the same material as the sides at the closed end. As with the open aviary, natural cover or a hiding box should be available so the bird can retire from view when you enter the aviary. Perches should not be too high, allowing plenty of head-room when the bird takes off and lands and the perches should be of varying thickness but not too thin for the species concerned (see *Initial Care and Symptoms, Diagnosis and Treatment*).

If neither of the above alternatives is possible, a clean clutter-free shed would offer the best alternative with the window barred as above. Although we would not recommend it for permanent accommodation, a raptor can live in a shed for a lengthy period with no apparent ill-effects, but be sure to provide regular bathing facilities.

Release

It is strongly urged that a raptor be released directly from the convalescent quarters. In this way, it has an orientation point where it can, and very often will, return for food in the initial difficult period of readjustment to the wild. Some rehabilitated raptors will continue to return sporadically for weeks or even months after release and they must always be sure of a meal if they do, so a keen lookout must be kept for their reappearance in the vicinity.

It is patently impossible to maintain a permanent watch for a returning bird but we found that, if we fed a patient at a regular time each day for the entire period of treatment and convalescence, it tended to reappear at about the same time of day after release. If there is any sign of it in the vicinity, food can then be placed on the roof of the aviary or shed or on the ledge of the release hatch, if one has been provided (see Fig. 11).

If the premises where the bird is being treated is not a desirable release point, we would suggest the bird be transferred elsewhere for its period of convalescence. Please do not simply take the bird somewhere and release it 'cold', no matter how quiet the spot chosen. Raptors have a hard enough row to hoe when released and many *need* that back-up of a place where they know food will be available.

Orphans

Finding a young bird apparently all alone is not sufficient reason for assuming it to be an orphan and carting it off home. In the case of a raptor, such a course might well result in a torn scalp or even a lost eye from the attack of an irate parent. There is, in fact, no easy formula for determining whether or not a particular infant has been abandoned but in general, we would advise leaving it where it is found and not touching it at all. This may seem rather callous but there is no doubt at all that the vast majority of *assumed* orphans are nothing of the sort.

. Of course, there are many circumstances in which youngsters simply must be rescued. For instance, most of our raptor chicks arrive as a result of tree felling which is just a bit much even for staunch tawny owl parents to countenance. In one recent season, we had no fewer than twenty-two newly hatched tawny owlets brought in during such operations, and most years produce at least a couple of families of one species or another.

Raptor infants are very easy to rear. As for the adults, we strongly recommend day-old chicks which must, of course, be chopped up and preferably dampened with water. The size of the pieces obviously depends on the species but you will find that a young raptor can swallow pieces much larger than you would imagine. During its first few weeks, indeed, it will eat much more than an adult of the same species, so keep on offering pieces until the bird has had enough. It will usually indicate this by holding the last piece in its beak for a time and then dropping it.

Offer food about four or five times a day and don't worry about set times. Owlets, for instance, will accept food and thrive just as well if fed during the day so there is no point in losing any sleep by feeding during the night.

If this sounds rather casual, that's because it is! For this group there is no need at all for a rigid regime or more frequent feeds. Raptors, even very young ones, are equipped to go without food for quite long periods which is quite logical if you give it some thought. All of their food has to be *caught*. In other words it is all very much alive and 'on the hoof', and not just waiting around to provide sustenance for madam raptor and family. Even on nice days (or nights) the collection of food is a chancy business (apart from a fair percentage of beetles which are somewhat easier to catch). Consider the problems on a foul, stormy day, of which we seem to get more than our fair share in this country, and you will appreciate why raptors and their offspring can manage – and indeed do manage – on a somewhat irregular diet.

At first, the youngster's beak may have to be opened and the pieces of food popped well in, either using blunt forceps or just with the fingers but most of them learn very quickly and will take hold of the food themselves when it is dangled before their beaks. If day-old chicks cannot be obtained and you have to use raw meat, add a sprinkling of bone meal to each feed and don't forget to add some kind of roughage – cat or dog hair, or even hair from an old spare wig or toupée, if you happen to use such adornments!

It is most difficult if you're only rearing a single youngster to avoid some measure of imprinting, but there are a few simple rules which should be rigidly adhered to if the bird is to have the optimum chance of surviving when released. The same rules apply of course if rearing more than one. Touch the bird or birds as little as possible. Never stroke or caress them in any way (some enjoy this, so it is a great temptation). Never talk to them. It's better (for them) at a later date that the sound of a human voice should frighten rather than encourage them.

As soon as the youngsters can feed themselves, try to prevent them seeing just where the food comes from. This is to try and stop the association of humans with food and may call for some ingenuity, depending on the set-up. In the early, hand-feeding stage, the chicks can be kept in a box, even a cardboard one, anywhere about the house and there is no need to provide artificial heat unless the ambient temperature drops very low (for the time of year). Our experience is that they will move away from artificial heat so, if in doubt, provide the heat but allow the opportunity to move away from it. By the way, do not provide bathing facilities until the youngsters change their down for feathers.

The remarks regarding pre-release and release of adult casualties apply also to hand-reared infants. In fact we consider quarters from which they can be released directly to be absolutely essential if the birds are to stand the optimum chance of survival. Feeding, too, should now be at a regular time (see *Release*).

There is a view quite commonly held that hand-reared raptors must be 'trained' to catch their food. We do not subscribe to this view. The so-called 'training' that some rearers believe in consists of introducing live mice to the aviary or pre-release quarters for the bird to kill and eat. We hold that this is not 'training' at all, but merely offering the bird an opportunity to exercise the predatory instincts it *already possesses*. *Of course* it must acquire skills in hunting but this sterile practise is no substitute for the real thing. The bird must acquire the necessary knowledge for survival *in the field* but with the back-up of an orientation point where food is available to supplement early inefficiency.

'That's all very well,' say the doubters, 'but how do you know your method works? How do you know that when the birds stop coming back for food they haven't just died?' Good and reasonable questions to which we would reply by quoting just one case (of many). The twenty-two tawny owlets mentioned earlier were all released from the same point at the same time and all were wearing BTO (British Trust for Ornithology) rings which made them easily identifiable. None were ever picked up, dead, dying or otherwise. Surely even the most sceptical must concede that if such a bunch had come to grief, at least one would have been recovered. By the way, one of this lot was still returning for an occasional meal two months after release!

Just when to effect the release is a rather difficult one. Most people who have successfully reared any wild creature are rather reluctant when it comes to the final step and this is quite understandable. It's a very harsh world out there. In the case of your young raptor or raptors, allow about four weeks *after* the birds are fully fledged and make the release during a settled spell of fine weather, preferably, or at least on a fine day. Diurnal species should be released in the early morning, nocturnal in the late evening (but while it is still light). If you have a release hatch, this is simply left open at feeding time. As with adult releases, have a good look around at this time each day after release, and don't stop doing so just because the bird has failed to appear for several days. Give it at least a fortnight from the last appearance before assuming it isn't coming back.

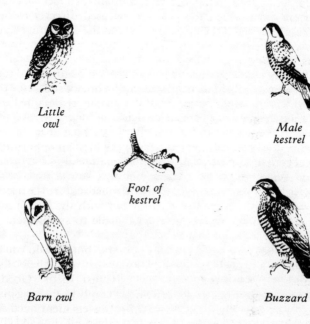

Little
owl

Male
kestrel

Foot of
kestrel

Barn owl

Buzzard

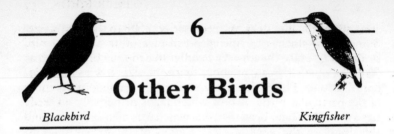

6

Other Birds

Blackbird   *Kingfisher*

This chapter may be considered too wide-ranging in that it deals with a very large number of species, but there are several reasons why we have lumped them all together. The first is that in spite of the wide variety of species included, they do have one thing in common, namely, they are all 'altricial', or 'nidiculous' (that is to say, birds which stay in the nest after hatching and are fed by the parents until fledged). The birds of prey of the previous chapter are, of course, also altricial, as are some of those in Chapters 2 and 3 and some which have traits of both altricial and precocial species but raptors are a somewhat specialist group, while those appearing in the other chapters fall more readily into the groups we have selected for them, rather than in this chapter.

A second reason is that although there are so many, and any of them *could* at some time appear as casualty or orphan, in practice very few do. Probably the main reason for this is that most of the species very sensibly conduct their affairs at a discreet distance from the human race. The principal casualties and orphans we have received from this group over the years are those commonly called 'garden birds' or others which do not fall strictly into this category but nonetheless live in close proximity to man. This is not to say that accidents and injuries do not happen to those living further afield, because they certainly do, but the incidence is undoubtedly much less where people are not involved, as are the chances of being rescued. One of these casualties is much more likely to make the next meal for some other creature on the lookout for just such a treat.

In silhouette, most of the group look very much alike, with all principal features modestly proportioned in relation to the bird's size. There are 'odd men out' such as the swift, the kingfisher, the rare hoopoe and one or two more, whose outlines look somewhat different. Size ranges from the raven at about 25in. (62.5cm) to the goldcrest at only 3½in. (9cm), and the grouping covers some ninety species.

Possible Handling Hazards

Most of this group will attempt to bite when handled and the strength of the bite does not necessarily relate to the bird's size. Some of the finches for instance can give quite a painful nip, sufficient to cause the unwary handler to drop the bird, whereas (say) the mistle thrush, at about twice the size, has a very mild, harmless bite. This is due in the main to the feeding preferences of the particular birds. A bird which feeds principally on seeds has a much stronger beak than one which eats mainly insects, and this leads to the general classification of the two groups as 'hardbills' and 'softbills'. The difference between the two can be appreciated when they have hold of your finger!

The raven has a formidable bite and is best handled with gloves. The other larger members of the crow family also have quite a strong bite but not usually sufficient to break the skin, while the smaller members do not have much of a bite but are apt to rap off a series of pecks with the sharp tip.

Although, apart from the raven, there is little or no danger of serious injury from a bird in this group, it is worth repeating the warning, *no bird should ever be held near the handler's face.*

Approach and Capture

The most general reaction from this group when approached is to escape, although some will try to hide at first and only break and flee at the last moment, when you are almost upon them. As the vast majority of the group are under 10in. (25cm) with a high proportion only half this length, they can be quite difficult to catch without exacerbating the injury and adding to the shock they will already be suffering.

A catching net (see Fig. 1 on page 7) is a positive boon for this job but if none is available, it is best to try and drop something over the bird. A coat is suitable for the larger species such as crows or wood-pigeons, but for the small birds, it should be something lightweight such as a towel or even a T-shirt. Alternatively, try trapping the bird under a cardboard box to which a pole or branch can be easily attached (Fig. 12), allowing the catching to be done without coming right up to the bird and causing it to flee.

Whatever you use to trap the bird, it should be removed very slowly until the bird can be grasped with its wings at its sides, then lowered slowly into the travelling container. Avoid rapid or jerky movements which will only cause panic, and try to support the feet during the move (when a bird doesn't feel its feet touching anything, it assumes it must be flying and will instinctively try to flap its wings).

Some of the crow family may 'have a go' at the container and the larger of them can certainly penetrate the average cardboard

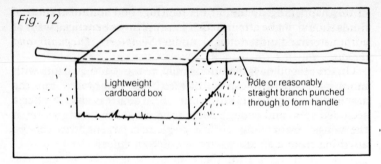

Fig. 12

Lightweight cardboard box

Pole or reasonably straight branch punched through to form handle

box with a little diligent work. But unless the journey is very long, and the bird is suffering only a minor injury which doesn't hinder its excavations, it is unlikely to make a large enough hole through which to escape before you reach your destination.

At the other end of the scale, some of the smaller birds can be carried in a paper bag (with air holes of course), with little danger of their escaping or even trying to. The general rule for this group is that they can be carried in anything large enough to contain them.

Initial Care

Rest, peace and quiet, and warmth are the first essentials. For the smaller species there are specially designed hospital cages which are quite good, but any kind of cage or box which can be covered to keep it quite dark will suffice for the first twenty-four hours. The airing cupboard is a good place to provide a nice warm ambient temperature, but even a covered hot water bottle near your patient is better than nothing. A temperature of around $25°C$ ($77°F$) should be aimed for, or even up to $30°C$ ($86°F$) if there is any way of grading the temperature, and the bird is sufficiently mobile to choose its own spot.

It is also desirable that the bird be given some fluid in these early stages. Warm water by itself is a great deal better than nothing, but if a pinch of glucose can be added, this will be most beneficial. An eye dropper can be used for this purpose but by far the best thing to use is a plastic syringe (without the needle of course). The actual quantity is not really critical, a few drops for a finch, and half a teaspoon (2ml) for a crow, repeated at about two-hourly intervals (but not during the night, when the bird should be left completely alone). The fluid is best administered at the hinge of the beak, a little at a time since care must be taken that none enters the glottis (which leads to the lungs). If the bird is allowed to breathe freely between drops, there is little danger of this happening. If the bird is panting, oral administration of fluids should not be attempted. There are more beneficial ways of administering fluids detailed under *Symptoms, Diagnosis and Treatment*.

On the second day, the bird should be moved to quarters with more light where it can be offered food and water, but the ambient temperature is still warm. The quarters should offer a secluded spot, and enough room to move around and to stretch the wings. Depending on the particular patient, this can be anything from a small cage to a whole room!

Food

Many are the weird and wonderful recipes for the feeding of wild birds in captivity and indeed, no stone should be left unturned in the effort to get your patient to eat. The turning of stones can be taken literally, by the way, since a good many of this group will appreciate a nice fat snail.

As mentioned earlier, most birds in this group are either insect-eaters or seed-eaters, or more likely a combination of both, with a preference for one or the other. Different beak shapes give a clue to this preference but virtually all cross the dividing line from time to time when something on the other side takes their fancy or when their preferred food is in short supply.

Insectivorous foods are available at pet shops, and softbills may also accept tinned dog or cat meat mixed with breadcrumbs, chopped-up bacon rind, cheese, finely chopped or minced raw meat, corned beef, plus any worms or snails which might be lurking about and even a few flies (but *not* those you've knocked off with a fly spray). Hardbills will in general accept food in captivity more readily than softbills, and can be given bread-crumbs, chopped greens and apple, plus budgie seed or indeed any other seed including grass seed (take care that it hasn't been dressed to repel birds). Most species in the group will accept chopped hard-boiled or scrambled egg, and many will readily accept a little fish such as tinned pilchards (in tomato sauce rather than oil).

The larger crows can do with rather more meat. Tinned dog meat will be acceptable but a dead day-old chick will be very much appreciated, as will any other meat or bones to pick at. A whole chicken or turkey carcase, after you've had your share, will be a veritable feast.

There are one or two specialists in the group who will require special catering. The woodpeckers and treecreepers should be provided with a nice thick (and preferably rotting) upright log, which they can explore for beetles and grubs. We have also had some success with these by plastering a mixture of insectivorous food and tinned dog meat onto the log. Kingfishers need small fish and we usually use whitebait for this species (see *Force-feeding*). Dried flies can *usually* be obtained from pet shops for flycatchers and these can be supplemented with any house or garden flies, a worm or two, and any grubs you can find. Folded leaves on trees and bushes often yield a rich harvest of grubs. For swifts, see *Force-feeding*.

We have not handled every species in this group – indeed it is doubtful if *anybody* has. It is easy to find out what any particular species eats in the wild since most bird books give you this information. Getting that same species to eat in captivity, when injured, is quite a different matter. Do not be afraid to experiment, for the bird is unlikely to voluntarily eat anything which will do it harm, and do not allow your patient's food preference in the wild to dominate your thinking. A bird which normally eats flies might quite easily enjoy a portion of plum pudding! Water should, of course, be provided for all. See also the notes about dishes and methods of presentation in the food section of Chapter 3.

Force-feeding

No animal (including ourselves) enjoys the experience of being forcibly fed, and if you couple this lack of enthusiasm for the actual operation with an abject fear of the creature doing it, this gives an indication of the bird's side of the matter. So don't force-feed birds in this group unless you are obliged to as a last resort.

Swifts will not normally feed themselves in captivity, but it is quite easy to force-feed them as they have mouths almost big enough to take a side of beef! Although they may be kept alive and may grow quite accustomed to a captive state (they appear to have little or no fear of humans) the chances of an injured swift being able to return to its singular mode of life are very slim indeed (see *Release*).

Uniformity of behaviour should not be expected, even with birds of the same species. Some kingfishers, for instance, will pick fish out of a bowl of water, others will grab and swallow a fish handed to them (head first), others will swallow a fish placed just in the beak (again head first) while still others will need to have the fish pushed down their throat.

Obviously you must be more selective when force-feeding to choose something near the bird's normal food range since it isn't taking the meal voluntarily, thereby making its own selection. A good starter, which will be satisfactory for most in this group, would be finely grated hard-boiled egg mixed with dampened breadcrumbs or scrambled egg by itself. The former can be made into pellets of a suitable size of the bird in question, the latter offered just in pieces.

The food may have to be placed well back on the tongue with the aid of blunt forceps and a good trick is to follow each piece with a drop or two of water from a syringe which will encourage the bird to swallow (see *Initial Care*).

Never try to open a beak by the tip, always near the hinge and always handle the beak very carefully to avoid the risk of distortion.

Symptoms, Diagnosis and Treatment

Injuries. The most frequent injury in this group is mauling by domestic cats, which causes shock and both internal and external injuries. Broken wings, broken legs and concussion caused by collision with cars or window panes are also fairly common. These accidents occur most commonly in the late spring and early summer when the youngsters are leaving the nest and are not very 'worldly wise'.

On examination the bird may show no external injuries, but it appears to be dead and is limp, both wings outspread and eyes closed. But when you pick it up, you can feel its heart still beating. Unfortunately many of them will not regain consciousness, especially those mauled by a cat, for this is a particularly traumatic experience for a little bird. Those that fly into a window pane or are hit by a car may recover provided the neck is not broken or extensive internal injuries caused. The simplest form of treatment is to place the bird in a little open box lined with tissue and put it in a dark quiet place until it has recovered. It is best to put the small box containing the unconscious bird inside a larger closed box or cage otherwise it may well recover and start flying at the windows, trying to get out of the room in which you have kept it. It can also be examined from time to time without stressing the bird which can easily be released when it has recovered.

Shock may be quite simply a loss of consciousness due to dissociation (a sort of blockage to the relay system) in the brain caused by a blow such as flying into a window. It is analogous to a knock-out in the boxing ring and normally the bird should recover. If the neck is broken, however, it will certainly die without regaining consciousness.

The shock caused by a cat-mauling is different. Dilation of the blood vessels – brought on by the mental anguish of being caught by a predator – causes a slowing of the heart rate and a fall in blood pressure. In nature this shock serves a very useful purpose because many prey animals caught by predators lose consciousness and thus are insensitive to the injuries subsequently inflicted. Death may occur because of the shock itself, or the bird may haemorrhage later.

The treatment for this form of shock is to increase the volume of the circulating blood by giving drugs that stimulate the heart and contract the blood vessels, or by giving fluids that will be absorbed into the blood system, also increasing its volume. The lay person can only give fluids by mouth provided the bird is able to swallow, and for this it must be conscious. Whereas the veterinary surgeon can give fluids by injection (or instruct a lay person) either into the vein, into the peritoneal cavity, or even under the skin, which will help to increase blood pressure and counteract the shock.

These injections are either blood replacers specially prepared for that purpose, or a 5 per cent solution of glucose sterilized for injection. Again, put the bird in a dry, not too warm, box in the dark and leave it alone for a quiet hour or so by which time it should have recovered. It is important not to disturb the bird too often once it has recovered. When it has recovered consciousness, if the injuries are slight, the bird can be released. But if it still appears to be weak then you should attempt to give it a small amount of fluid containing glucose (at about 1 per cent concentration – roughly a heaped teaspoon to 1pt (600ml) water). A bird should *never* be released to the wild until it is strong and fit enough to fly, otherwise it will be subject to attack by ground predators and may not survive.

Sometimes the brain is damaged, usually by a haemorrhage or blood clot in the nervous tissue. Symptoms are a partial paralysis of one side of the bird, or of a wing or limb, or a circling movement where the bird continually flutters or staggers round with its head bent in the direction of the circling. Prognosis is bad and it is kinder to put the bird to sleep if it shows no improvement in twenty-four hours. Broken wings and legs are not uncommon but because many of these birds do not rely on *perfect* flight to obtain their food, being mainly seed and insect eaters, it is possible for them to get about perfectly well with a slightly crooked wing or leg and some can manage with only one leg.

Diseases and Poisoning. Poisoning can occur from time to time due to the accidental contamination of the plants upon which these birds feed with insecticides. Fruit tree and garden sprays and some agricultural sprays are particularly hazardous and cases have been reported where a number of small birds have been found dead. Always use any spray very carefully to minimize the ever-present risk. Little can be done with this kind of poisoning even if the birds are found alive. There is no specific antidote and careful nursing is the only treatment. It is usually too late to administer fluids to wash out the poisons, which are very rapidly absorbed.

Symptoms of disease in birds are of such a general nature that they seem to apply to a number of diseases. More often than not diagnosis cannot be made on symptoms alone. But many species of these garden birds are susceptible to the common bird diseases. Psittacosis in its chronic form is particularly prevalent in birds such as sparrows and pigeons. Tuberculosis can affect wood-pigeons, sparrows and starlings, and salmonellosis has been found in pigeons and rooks. As is the case with most wild creatures, the symptoms are not evident until either the disease is advanced and little can be done, or until the animal is shocked or stressed by some other catastrophe which precipitates the acute form of the disease, and rapid death.

Nearly every wild creature, bird or mammal, carries internal and external parasites, but provided the bird is living a natural life with a reasonable amount of food no untoward effects can be seen. Should food supplies diminish, water supplies dry up in a drought season, or there is a severe winter, disease symptoms may become manifest and they usually progress rapidly to death.

If a conscious wild bird can be picked up fairly readily, you can be certain that there is something seriously wrong with it. If there are no signs of injury then it is quite likely to be suffering from disease. Diagnosis is difficult for the veterinary surgeon and almost impossible for the layman. Treatment will be almost useless for the individual bird because it may have been hiding the symptoms of the disease for some time before it became ill.

The best treatment for these cases is to keep the bird warm (approximately 25°C, 77°F) and provide it with a plentiful supply of the correct food and water. If it is suffering from a disease that is far advanced then it will die fairly quickly. If not, there is a good chance that it will recover and once able to fly it may be released.

Two examples that are fairly typical of an ordinary member of the public being involved with wild bird care, one with a happy ending, the other not, show the vicissitudes of nature. In the middle of a very bad winter, a young man found the smallest of British birds, the goldcrest, sitting outside a greenhouse looking cold and dejected. It was fairly easy to open the greenhouse door and slowly and carefully drive the little fellow inside. A frantic search was then made for some insects for the bird to eat and a few were found. These were offered on a saucer and readily taken. The bird then began hopping about, in the course of which it hopped onto his shoe and cocked an eye up at him. There were high hopes that it would recover and everyone searched for more insects and brought a heater in to warm the greenhouse. The goldcrest fed until it was dark, but, because it was mid-winter, darkness came early and the night was long. The next day it was found dead, causing much sadness and disappointment. And no obvious cause as to the reason why the bird died.

On another occasion a blackbird was taken to a vet for treatment with a badly smashed wing. Both the radius and ulna had been broken in more than one place and the wing flopped about loosely. The skin was broken on the inside and it had been bleeding. But the bird was not shocked, seeming to accept its human companions, and would eat food offered in the hand. The wing was treated and then strapped to the bird's body. Thereafter careful nursing by the lady who found it effected a complete recovery, for when she brought it back and the strapping was removed, it flew about the room almost normally. She kept it a few more days and then finally released it into the garden and was delighted when it used to return each day to her bird table to be fed from her hand. One bird at least had learned that mankind need not always be feared.

General Care

The plumage of many of this group is apt to deteriorate and/or become badly soiled if the bird is kept indoors for very long, so it is strongly recommended that your patient be moved out of doors as soon as possible where the plumage can 'weather' normally. If you cannot provide a suitable aviary yourself, do not be possessive, but pass the bird on to someone who can.

Most of the smaller members of this group will benefit in convalescence from the reassuring presence of other birds about them, albeit of other species. They will fare quite happily in an aviary of budgies, foreign finches or even some of the smaller parakeets (although care and sound advice must be taken with the latter since some species of parakeet are rather pugnacious). We keep a number of resident budgies in our aviaries specifically to fulfill this therapeutic function.

Crows can be kept with other members of the same family or

with any other birds large enough to 'hold their own' such as pheasants, although it might be judicious to keep ravens on their own.

The field is wide if you are intending to build your own aviary but one or two points should always be incorporated. Never place the aviary in such a way that people can walk all round it. This is very traumatic for a bird, even one accustomed to being in an aviary, as such conditions may completely deprive it of its flight line (the distance at which a bird feels safe from a human). Allow sufficient head-room. It is important when you enter the aviary that the bird should be able either to hide, or get above your head (allow 7 feet or at least 2 metres minimum). Allow a bit of cover from heavy rain (PVC sheeting for example), but do not cover the whole top with solid material. Within the limits of the materials available, increase the length at the expense of the width. In other words a long rectangle is preferable to a square, providing you only allow people to approach at one end and not walk around the sides too. This will enhance the flight line which will add to the bird's peace of mind and assist recuperation. A grass base is preferable for all of this group although you will have to introduce sand or gravel at favourite sitting spots as the grass becomes soiled with droppings.

Release

With about ninety species in the group, it is difficult to generalize as to how and where release should be effected. As with the shearwaters mentioned in Chapter 2, some birds thought to be casualties are merely birds which have inadvertently become grounded and cannot take off from flat ground. The swift is such a bird, with swallows and martins also suffering from the same problem to some extent. Such a grounded bird may only need a boost into the air in order to be on its way.

The trouble with releasing rehabilitated casualties of this group from an urban aviary is that you can never be quite sure what the bird will do when released. It may fly away rapidly on release, and may well reach a suitable habitat under its own steam, long before you could reach the same spot by car. On the other hand, a 'country' bird released from an aviary in the middle of a city may find some difficulty in orientating itself and may fall easy prey for a cat. On balance, it is probably best to take the bird to an area best suited to its species and most bird books will furnish you with this knowledge.

The bird books will also tell you whether your bird is a resident or migratory species and if the latter, should it have already left the country? You may have to consider keeping the bird until the following spring and this can certainly be done although we can only claim personal experience with a grasshopper warbler which spent a winter quite happily in an outdoor aviary (with a house) and in reverse, a fieldfare (a winter visitor) which spent a summer with us.

Orphans

Nestlings can come to hand in a variety of ways but the most common is someone chopping down a tree or taking the roof off a building at the wrong time. If there is any possibility of the nest being saved *in situ*, this should be done since the parents will almost certainly continue feeding the family if given a reasonable opportunity to do so. In many cases this simply isn't possible, and hand-rearing has to be undertaken. Fortunately, the nestlings of this group all gape for their food and it is a fairly easy, if arduous, task to feed them. Most will open their beaks at the slightest sound of any sort, some will only open up at a slight tap on the edge of the nest or if you make a soft, hissing sound.

In the circumstances described above, it may be possible to rescue the nest as well as the nestlings, in which case they should continue to live in it. If the nest has been destroyed, one must be constructed which resembles the original as closely as possible – which means round in shape, small enough to keep the youngsters close together, and with sides high enough to stop them falling out. A round container ranging from the bottom of a plastic washing-up liquid bottle to a biscuit tin, depending on the species, lined with paper kitchen towels, should prove satisfactory. It is not advisable to use an old nest as this may contain some undesirable residents.

The nestlings will require warmth, at least until they get their feathers, and thereafter at nights until they leave the nest. A temperature in the region of 30°C (86°F) is necessary, but since these infants cannot move away if too hot, take some trouble over the placing of the heat source and keep a close eye on the reaction of the infants. An infra-red lamp placed at a certain height over the nest may be just right during the night but may rapidly get too hot on a very warm day. In too high a temperature, the infants will be making obvious efforts to move away from each other with necks stretched out. They may pant as well. When too cold, their bodies will feel cold to the touch.

A bit of thought should also be given as to where the nest is placed. The reason for this is that the youngsters should remain in the same quarters until they are feeding themselves and they will want to be out of the nest and hopping about before then. So, if when they start leaving the nest, they are immediately moved somewhere else – to an aviary, perhaps – they may panic in the new surroundings when approached and fail to come for food. If they are kept in the same room as the nest, this is unlikely to arise and they will continue to gape for the person who has reared them (although they may not for a stranger).

In the wild all these nestlings, including the seed eaters, are fed largely on insects, and we have found a mixture of insectivorous food and dampened breadcrumbs to be satisfactory for most. Very young birds of the smaller species (e.g. tits) are usually started on sieved hard-boiled egg yolk, mixed to a paste with a little water and served with a small artist's paint brush. Crushed biscuit can be added to the egg yolk (which mixture can be obtained commercially) for slightly larger youngsters.

When using the insect/breadcrumb formula, the mixture should be firm enough to make into pellets which will vary in size according to species. A finch will take pellets about $\frac{1}{2}$in. long by $\frac{1}{8}$in. diameter (125×25mm) while a crow will comfortably manage 1in. long by $\frac{1}{2}$in. diameter (250×125mm). To save giving water separately as well as helping them to go down easily, dip each pellet in water just before giving it to the bird.

'Bald' infants should be fed every hour from dawn till dusk and give them as much as they will take at each feed. It is impossible to overfeed nestlings as they will stop gaping when they have had enough each time, and this is a big help in sorting out just who has been fed when there are several in the nest. They will also defaecate after a feed and as the dropping is covered with a fine skin, it can be picked up from the nest with a pair of tweezers before it makes a mess of both nest and birds – although we do not advocate swallowing it, as the parent birds frequently do!

The nestlings will grow very rapidly and will soon be clambering up onto the sides of the nest. The length of time they will need to be hand-fed is very difficult to define exactly (even within a species), for most are still fed by their parents for some time after leaving the nest. As soon as the youngsters begin to get around, leave some of the same food in the vicinity for them to peck at, which they will do very inefficiently at first, and gradually cut down the number of feeds to four a day. This should be maintained until they are fully self-sufficient, when most will cease to beg for food at your approach. The crow family are particularly difficult to break off. They should continue to be hand-fed for at least two weeks after leaving the nest and whatever they manage to pick up themselves will need to be supplemented for about another two, after which hand-feeds should be few and far between to encourage them to fend for themselves.

All too frequently, people pick up fledglings which have fallen a few days prematurely from the nest, or which have recently vacated it. These are a vastly different proposition to nestlings and as a general rule, should be left where they are found. The parents will almost certainly continue to feed the youngster and will make a much better job of it than the finder is likely to do. The problem is that it is most difficult to make such a decision in any given circumstances and it is quite impossible to generalize. Take the case of an almost fledged bird which has managed to fall out of a nest in an urban area. Even if the parents do continue to feed it, the chances are that it will fall prey to one of the many cats which doubtless prowl the neighbourhood. Knowing the location of the nest, it might seem like a good idea to climb up and put the youngster back, but to do so would almost certainly cause the others to explode from the nest in panic, thereby making the problem much worse.

The best course in such circumstances is to place the youngster in a box which it cannot easily jump out of but which affords access for the parents, and place the box in a sheltered position off the ground near the nest but without disturbing it. The parents will almost certainly find the youngster and continue to feed it. You can in any case keep watch from a distance to ensure that they do, and the youngster can follow the parents out when it is fully fledged. Ordinary bird cages have frequently been used for this purpose and the parents have continued to feed the caged youngster through the bars, even when the cage is taken indoors at night and put out only through the day. In this case, the youngster has to be released manually, when judged ready.

There are undoubtedly many cases where the only recourse is to attempt the rearing of a fledgling but it is much more difficult than rearing from the nestling stage and should not be lightly undertaken. The problem is that a bird's innate fear of humans is already manifest by the fledgling stage but it is not yet ready to feed itself. Each feed is, therefore, a struggle between hunger and terror with the bird having to be caught and held and force-fed each time. Not the best of starts, and one that often ends in disaster with the bird dying. If you are obliged for any reason to try it, the notes on force-feeding adults apply (see page 60).

It is difficult to give any hard and fast rules regarding the release of hand-reared youngsters of this group. You must not release them prematurely, but you must release them in plenty of time to prepare for migration if of a migratory species, and you must release in time to ensure a reasonable period of complete self-sufficiency before winter sets in if a resident species. The optimum time is early to mid summer, when nature intended anyway. Occasionally, a bird of this group will stay in the vicinity after release in which case you can continue to provide food, but most will leave immediately.

Blue tit

Great tit

Long-tailed tit

Green woodpecker

Nestlings gaping for food

Crow

Song thrush

Swallow

Wood-pigeon

Goldcrest

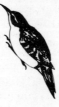

Tree creeper

Chaffinch

7

Oil Pollution

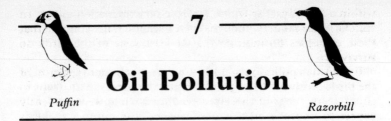

Puffin

Razorbill

In the field of cleaning and rehabilitating birds contaminated with oil, there are quite a number of people who 'know how to do it' and indeed some do perform a very good job. Unfortunately, many don't, and they bring the whole endeavour into disrepute, an endeavour which already suffers from a distinct lack of credibility in many quarters. A number of critics flatly refuse to believe that a bird can be returned to 100 per cent buoyancy after cleaning. Others say that even if it can be done, the birds do not survive after being returned to the sea, and even more claim the whole exercise is of no significance anyway, due to the very small numbers which can be saved from any incident. We have been engaged in this work for a number of years, using methods devised originally by the Zoology Department of Newcastle University, and can claim to have achieved some success in answering the doubters.

In the case of birds contaminated with most crude oils we can, without any reservation, achieve a return to 100 per cent buoyancy (that is, where no water can penetrate the feathers) in a period measured only in days. This we have demonstrated to many who doubted it could be done. Long-term survival is much more difficult to prove, relying as it does on birds being picked up again after return to sea which, of course can only happen when the bird is once more in difficulties of some sort. In other words, a bird which has returned to a normal life is unlikely to be picked up again, which applies particularly to sea-going birds like auks.

Of the many birds we have cleaned and released, only three – all guillemots – have been subsequently found again. One released off the Yorkshire coast was picked up six months later in Holland, still alive but with an injured leg. One released off the Yorkshire coast was picked up near the same spot (its home breeding ground) two years and one month later having just died. A third released off the Dorset coast and picked up in Eire, two years and four months later, was re-oiled but still alive.

We must admit that from most batches of birds released, there are almost invariably a small number that float in dead or dying within a few days, for which we have no explanation as yet. In spite of these failures, though, even a sceptic must concede that these examples do indicate that at least *some* of the birds do survive.

From small pollution incidents, we can put back to sea most of the birds received. In larger incidents, the success rate drops to about 50 per cent of those received, and while we confidently expect to improve on this performance, the number of birds saved from any major incident is likely to remain comparatively small in relation to the total number involved. Which brings us to the third point of objection – is it worth doing at all? To answer this, we would quote Dr Perrins of Oxford, writing about auks on islands off the Welsh coast: 'For species whose recruitment seems to be only marginally sufficient to replace the losses of breeding adults, even small reductions in such mortality might be critical if the populations are to survive' ('Life Tables for Auks', *Ibis*, 120, pp 128–9).

The birds principally affected by oil spills at sea are the auks, members of which family include the guillemot, the razorbill and the puffin. Depending on where the spill occurs, other species can also be affected such as divers, sea ducks, grebes, gannets, etc., but very nearly every incident includes auks and they are usually the principal sufferers.

In addition to spills at sea, there are also more than enough river and estuary incidents. In these, the principal victims are mute swans and mallard ducks although quite a number of other species can be involved.

Mammals can also be caught up in oiling incidents, notably seals, but there have been cases of otters being affected and even sheep, though the involvement of mammals is usually minimal, which is just as well. But since they are by far the greatest sufferers, this chapter will be devoted to birds, although the *principles* of cleaning apply equally to any oiled mammal which may be encountered. Obviously the actual *methods* used to achieve the end result may need considerable modification to accommodate the species concerned. It would be rather difficult to get a large, irate bull seal into a bowl of water!

Possible Handling Hazards
The details in Chapters 1, 2 and 3 apply equally here. Obviously, if large numbers of birds are to be collected, it would be a sensible move to wear a pair of gloves both to protect the hands from bites and to save getting them covered in oil. Overalls and wellington boots are a good idea too.

Approach and Capture

In large-scale operations, there will almost certainly be an organized team doing the collection but it is by no means unusual for an individual bird to be found by an individual person, particularly after a bad storm, in which case the notes in Chapter 2 would apply, bearing in mind that anything you cover the bird with may well be ruined by the oil.

Transportation

Contrary to what many people think, oiled birds can be carried for long distances with no apparent ill-effects providing they are not overcrowded and are carried in an enclosed vehicle. It is our contention that to a bird, standing in a moving vehicle is no different to standing in a static situation. It has no conception of 'a vehicle' and consequently suffers no more stress from being in one than from being in any other situation outside its normal experience. We have received birds which have been on the road for periods up to ten hours and the birds have arrived in much better condition than the drivers of the vehicles!

Cardboard 'pet carrier' containers are ideal for auks, with no more than four in one which is roughly 18 × 12 × 12in. (45 × 30 × 30cm). Other species such as ducks and divers can also be carried in these same boxes but only one or possibly two to a box. Even gannets have been carried in the same sized boxes with no apparent ill-effects but we would recommend rather larger containers – cardboard boxes – for this large species.

After a great deal of experience, we have dispensed with the practice of covering each bird with a 'poncho' or a covering with a hole for the head, having found that it can be dangerous to the birds and is of little value anyway. The idea was to prevent preening and consequent further ingestion of oil but we have found that most seabirds do very little preening once they are out of sight of water and the little they do is half-hearted and ineffectual. If an auk should fall over, as they are apt to do while wearing a poncho, it is usually quite unable to regain its feet and is consequently likely to be trampled on or fallen onto by the others. Tubular bandages and even socks have been used on occasion to totally immobilize birds, as well as keep them warm. Such wrappings certainly achieve total immobilization but we have found that, far from keeping the birds warm, they appeared to have the effect of actually *lowering* the bird's body temperature. In incidents where birds have been sent to us wearing ponchos or other coverings, en route mortality has been over 20 per cent. In incidents where they have been sent without such coverings, under 5 per cent.

Initial Care

As well as depriving a bird of buoyancy, oil also impairs the insulating qualities of the plumage and since, for several reasons, most oiling incidents occur in the winter, the first essential is to provide a warm room in which to house the birds. And since they will, in all probability, have been without food for several days, a good meal is the second essential. We also begin a short course of medication as soon as possible after capture which is one-quarter tablet of Kaobiotic (available from Upjohn Ltd) twice a day for a maximum of seven days for a bird of auk size.

The floor of the room or pen should be covered with thick newspaper or cloth and this should be changed regularly to prevent further contamination with the bird's own faeces. Do *not* use hay, straw, or similar covering (see *Symptoms, Diagnosis and Treatment*, this chapter, also Chapter 2, *Initial Care*).

Food

The type of food offered obviously depends on the species involved, and for a guide to this, refer to the food sections of Chapters 1, 2 or 3.

Force-feeding

Most seabirds will accept food readily, if not from a dish, then thrown down in front of them. If your bird fails to eat, the best course is to slip it some food when administering its medication although it should be noted that a seabird which does not feed itself from the start, seldom makes it back to sea (although you can keep such a bird alive in captivity virtually indefinitely). For methods of force-feeding, refer to the appropriate chapter for the species.

Symptoms, Diagnosis and Treatment

As mentioned in previous chapters, many wild birds and animals are infested with parasites, both internally and externally, and often infected by diseases that produce no symptoms unless the animal is stressed or physically below par.

Enteritis is another problem when the birds are first picked up. It may be caused by the stress, but it may also be caused, of course, by ingestion of oil. At any rate, as already described, the bird is treated with an antibiotic mixture at the very beginning, and should enteritis flare up during the subsequent recovery period, further treatments may be given.

Aspergillosis has been found in many species of birds from different habitats, but mainly in temperate zones. The cause is a fungus which grows in the lungs and air sacs of the bird and the symptoms produced when the disease is advanced are respiratory. The bird breathes with its beak open and produces a rattling sound. It is thought to be a major cause of death in herring gulls and mallards and the source of infection is believed to be mouldy food material and bedding, particularly hay and straw. Though it is a very common disease of penguins in captivity no naturally occurring case has been found in wild penguins in the Antarctic. It is obviously a disease caused and certainly exacerbated by stress and overcrowding.

The common lesions found on post-mortem examination are small circumscribed yellow nodules varying from the size of a pin head to a few centimetres in diameter. They are found in the lungs and air sacs, sometimes in the trachea, and occasionally in other organs as well. The disease is spread by the spores which are coughed up or excreted which contaminate the food and can remain viable for a long period of time. Therefore, it is important to keep these wild birds on clean disinfected standing (such as concrete), on clean dry newspaper, and in a building free from dust, cobwebs etc. Unfortunately to date there is no treatment for this disease.

Staphylococcal infection of the legs, which produces swaying of the joints and an inability to walk properly, is relatively common amongst wild birds that are kept on a hard standing for any length of time. This was particularly hazardous in the early days of treatment when birds were kept on concrete for long periods before being released. Nowadays the period of treatment has been very much reduced, and the birds can be got into a buoyant state allowing release in a very much shorter time. This reduces the susceptibility to staphylococcal infection. Nevertheless, it does occur from time to time and can be arrested by treatment with a broad-spectrum antibiotic such as Oxytetracyclin. However, once it is well established in the bird it is almost impossible to cure completely. Prevention, therefore, must be the main aim, and to this end keep the birds a minimum length of time in captivity, and make sure that the areas where they are kept are as clean and sterile as possible. Newspapers are in plentiful supply, unlikely to carry any infections and make an excellent floor covering – but do replace them frequently.

General Care (including Cleaning)

Although it is easy to describe how to clean birds, in practice it is a highly skilled, meticulous operation and we do *not* recommend people trying it themselves. Knowing *how* to do it is not enough, as a period of training is essential. In fact we would say with virtual certainty that anyone trying it just from written instructions would have about as much chance of success as someone learning to drive a car by the same means.

Many processed oils are much more intractable than crude and are more difficult, or in some cases even impossible, to remove successfully. Heavy solvents should never be resorted to since the vapours exuded can kill the birds (which rather defeats the object). Occasionally, it may be necessary to retain birds for lengthy periods to let the oil simply 'weather off'. This can be done with some species such as ducks or swans, but should not be attempted with ocean species such as auks which become conditioned to human presence very easily. If these species are contaminated with a type of oil which does not yield to detergents, we would recommend they be destroyed. The only alternatives are to put them back to sea less than adequately cleaned to face a lingering death or to keep them permanently in captivity (see Appendix A on the law).

When we receive oiled birds, we go about treatment in the following way. We leave the bird to be cleaned for about two or three days after its arrival – even longer if it appears in poor condition. A fit bird has a nice round, bright eye and this is the most obvious sign to look for in choosing a bird for cleaning.

A constant flow of water at high pressure and at 40°C (104°F) is absolutely essential to the cleaning process. *If this basic requirement is not available, there is no point whatsoever in attempting to clean birds.* Other desirable equipment includes a large sink, a supply of household washing-up liquid (effective for most crude oils) and a further room or pen where the birds can be placed after cleaning, prior to moving them out of doors. The water supply should be equipped with a hand-held shower attachment, and there should be two people to work as a team for each bird.

Make up a solution of washing-up liquid in a bowl of hot water (40 C, 104 F) to a strength of about 2 per cent (approximately half a cup to a large washing-up bowl of hot water). The person holding should hold the bird in the water up to its neck and the person cleaning should work the solution well into the plumage, paying particular attention to the head and neck. It is wise to secure the beak with a rubber band or something similar to save wear and tear on the hands! When the solution has been well worked into the head, back and tops of wings, the bird must be turned over and the breast, flanks and under wings attended to. Several changes of water and cleaning solution will be necessary during this process and it may be that the bird will need more than one wash to remove all the oil, in which case two or three days should elapse between 'sessions'. Every trace of oil both on the surface and under the plumage must be removed. Most plumage can be quite vigorously agitated with no ill-effects. Providing the centre quill of a feather is not broken, the bird will 'zip up' the disturbed barbs (the narrow strips to either side of the centre quill forming the feather itself) quite easily, as well as rearranging the complete infrastructure of the plumage, during subsequent preening. Gentleness is *not* synonymous with kindness in this operation.

When all the oil has been removed, the bird should be sprayed with the shower, again at 40°C (104°F), jetting the water strongly into the plumage against the lay of the feathers so that it penetrates to the skin. This all-important part of the cleaning process should continue until the water 'beads off' rather than soaking in and this state must be achieved for the whole of the plumage. The water beads off when all the detergent has been removed and the feathers return to their normal state. (It is the delicate intricate structure of the feather rather than preen gland wax, that gives it water-repellency, and therefore the bird buoyancy). The spraying should be done systematically – head, neck, back, tops of wings, then over for breast, flanks and under wings. During the rinsing operations the bird must be carefully held to ensure that detergent residues do not affect areas already cleaned. Once completely cleared of residues, the bird should be virtually dry although the wings and tail of some species such as cormorants are not 100 per cent waterproof and will remain wet after the cleaning process. If the job has been done properly, it should not be necessary to *dry* the bird and it should not, at this stage, be wrapped in a cloth. Place the bird in a clean warm room or pen (obviously *not* the one it was using previously) and leave it alone to preen. Provide some food as most birds appear to be ready for a snack immediately after cleaning. Do not, at this stage, use newspaper on the floor as the printers ink may cause a bit of contamination of its own which was not obvious or critical before. Do not use cloth either as there is every likelihood it will contain residues of the detergent it was washed in which may get onto the feathers. Absorbent paper towels are ideal for the floor at this stage but may be prohibitive in price if a lot of birds are to be catered for, in which case the floor may have to be left bare. The birds will only be here for one night, though, and should be able to go to an outside pool the following day. If the job has been done properly, *they should be completely buoyant.*

The outside paddock in which the birds are housed prior to release must be kept as clean as possible. For auks, smooth concrete is preferable. For others such as waterfowl, grass is satisfactory although this very quickly becomes contaminated with the bird's faeces if the area is small. Whatever kind of pool is used, it must have its water changed and sediments cleaned out at least once a day. There should also be a facility for keeping up a constant flow, skimming the surface and preventing the build-up of a surface film on the water which may affect the bird's plumage, leading to a further loss of buoyancy.

Waterfowl need as much ground area as can be allocated, in addition to the pool. Auks need very little 'walking space' and their activities are best confined to a narrow ledge, no more than a foot wide, around the pool, which can be improvised in a number of ways – timber or concrete blocks covered with polythene sheeting for instance. Auks also prefer a blank wall to stand against as they do on the cliff face.

Do not put fish into the pool for, although it is nice to see the birds diving for them, oil from the fish contributes greatly to the build-up of a surface film in a small area.

Release

A buoyancy test must be carried out prior to release in which the birds are compelled to remain in the pool for a minimum of twenty minutes, by which time any deficiencies in their buoyancy will become apparent. It is not enough to simply observe the birds pottering about and jumping in and out of the pool of their own volition, when they can look excellent and apparently perfect. Confinement to the water tells a different story, when water can slowly 'leak' through even one small patch. The bird will begin to exhibit signs of this by spreading its wings on the surface and flapping in an endeavour to correct flotation level.

After the twenty-minute test, each bird should be examined minutely and should be *completely dry* (but see the page opposite about cormorants). If it passes this test and is also in good physical condition, it is ready to be released. *But a bird should never be released if it has even a small damp patch as it will most certainly perish.* In *optimum* circumstances, release can be as little as a week after capture. In practice, it usually works out a little longer but release should be effected as soon as possible.

In oiling cases, it would be silly to take the birds back where they came from, if there is a probability of oil still hanging around, and it is not necessary to do so. They can be released from any quiet stretch of coast.

PART TWO
MAMMALS

8

Small ones

We are making a rather sweeping generalization here by lumping this group together in spite of their differences – as we did in Chapter 6. In this case, though, we are dealing with around fifteen species only, as opposed to the ninety or so birds we discussed then.

The group ranges in size from the brown rat (or common rat) – which can be about 10in. (25cm) long plus a tail of perhaps another 8in. (20cm) – to the pigmy shrew at about 2¼in. (5.75cm) plus 1½in. (3.75cm) of tail. Apart from the mole which has quite a distinctive appearance, the group do bear a superficial resemblance to one another in that they could all be described as 'small furry animals' – and this is about as much as many people would wish to know about them!

Most people would be able to identify a rat, brown or black, before they *and* the rat made a rapid departure from one another, but the others we deal with in this chapter are more difficult to tell apart. To the average town dweller, all small furry animals, if they aren't large enough to be rats, are mice whereas there are in fact three groups. The shrews have a very pointed muzzle, small ears which can hardly be seen, and fairly short tails. Mice too have pointed muzzles (but nothing like as long as the shrews), but have ears which are fairly prominent and longish tails. The third group, the voles, have inconspicuous ears and shortish tails (like the shrews), but blunt noses.

The odd men out in the group are the dormouse and the edible dormouse, which look like tiny squirrels, and the mole, which has a beautiful coat resembling velvet, and front feet that appear to belong to a much larger animal. The fur of the mole is interesting in that it will lie in any direction – with most mammals it only lies pointing to the rear. The poor old mole is a creature that suffers much more punishment than his crime really warrants. Although it must be admitted that it *looks* unsightly, most of the damage done by the offender is of a very superficial nature which, in a court of law, would call for a modest fine – not a prison sentence, and most certainly not the death sentence.

On the other hand rats, both brown and black, and the house mouse, if not kept under rigid control, could conceivably become strong rivals for very existence with the human race. They are overwhelmingly prolific, are sexually mature at a very early age (rats at three months, mice at only six weeks) producing anything up to thirty-five to forty young per year. Some simple mathematics will give an indication of just how breathtaking this recruitment rate is. They will eat prodigious quantities of virtually anything edible and will destroy much more by fouling. Rats in particular are very bright, not easily trapped, and they live anywhere and everywhere we do, doing extensive damage both to food supplies and to property.

Although people in general are unaware of it, the human race is at constant war with these animals and we aren't winning the war, only managing to hold our own. If we get down to basics, we are engaged in the same activity as every other species on earth – namely, the struggle for survival. We can live in peaceful co-existence with most species, but with some, tolerance and benevolence become luxuries which threaten our own species and as such, simply cannot be afforded. Such a conflict of fundamental interests has always existed and will always exist between rats and house mice on the one hand and ourselves on the other.

As to the others in the group, shrews are harmless and indeed useful in that they eat snails and insects. The remainder *can* cause varying amounts of agricultural and/or forestry damage, depending on the density of a particular species in a particular area. In general, their numbers are kept in check by a variety of predators including foxes, various birds of prey, stoats, weasels as well as domestic cats. Also, the life span of most is fleeting, by our standards, some as little as twelve to eighteen months.

It is very seldom a casualty of this group will come to hand in that the principal cause of injury is attack by predators, and this is almost invariably fatal. As the reason for the attack is to provide a meal for said predator (or offspring) the carcases are not left lying around, so it is seldom one comes across even a dead one. The only real exceptions to this are 'things the cat dragged in' and even these, if still alive, are likely to be suffering severe shock and injuries from which they will not recover.

There are certain of the group, namely rats and house mice, which we could not possibly recommend treating, even if anyone should wish to do so. There are points at which compassion becomes fanaticism and this is one of them. It *is* possible to keep a rat or a house mouse as a pet. Domestic varieties of both are widely kept, although in the main for experimental purposes, which is yet another subject and no part of this book. We do not recommend the keeping of the wild varieties as pets since a single one would lead a life of utter frustration in such circumstances.

Moles are brought to us occasionally after being caught by cats, and the odd dormouse will be raked out of hibernation by a gardener. Many others are taken out of hibernation by predators and eaten. It is estimated that at least three quarters of all dormice die this way. A common shrew can be rescued from a cat still alive, because although cats catch and kill these harmless and beneficial animals in large numbers, ironically they won't eat them. The only other casualties of the group we can recall from the past ten years or so are one bank vole and two long-tailed fieldmice, and this probably reflects the public's feelings toward the group as a whole. As mentioned earlier, to most people all small furry creatures are mice (meaning house mice) and as such, are more likely to be killed than rescued. Since this is our own view in the case of house mice we can't really complain if a person who doesn't know the difference, hits first and asks questions afterwards. But it is a pity that the harmless ones suffer the same fate as well.

Possible Handling Hazards

Most of the group can and will bite, and apart from any injury caused by the actual bite itself, there may be other complications. The bite of the water shrew is said to be poisonous and others can be 'carriers' (see *Symptoms, Diagnosis and Treatment*). The exception is the dormouse which will show no inclination to bite at all. It is one of the very few 'tame' wild animals showing no fear of humans and indeed exhibits only a friendly interest in anyone handling it. On one occasion a dormouse was brought in to us, and we could find nothing wrong with it. An assistant was instructed to take it into one of the paddocks out of harm's way, where it could go or stay as it wished. The assistant returned a few moments later, having carried out the instructions, with the dormouse skipping along behind him!

Approach and Capture

All the group are very agile and, in the open, very difficult to catch if still mobile – except the dormouse which will give itself up! Even in a confined space, their quick, darting movements are quite unpredictable. Trapping under a jam-jar is about the best method of capture, and you can then see through the glass just what it is you have caught – a mouse, a shrew or a vole. The exact species doesn't particularly matter at this stage. Obviously a rat will not fit under a jam-jar and if one needs to be caught rather than killed, a coat should be thrown over it. It will prefer to stay under the coat in the dark than venture out in the open again. There are many reliably witnessed instances of rats attacking people but the persons concerned are either dead, incapacitated or are babies. The stories of cornered rats leaping for the throat of the person doing the cornering are somewhat more difficult to authenticate, and are at best doubtful. In our experience, all of a rat's efforts are concentrated in trying to find a hiding place, with none left over for a counter-attack on the pursuer. If you feel the slightest revulsion or fear, it is best you do not even attempt to catch a rat.

Transportation

If it should be necessary to transport the rat you have caught, wrap it up slowly and carefully in the coat you have covered it with then drop it and the coat into a sack and tie the neck. The rat could, of course, chew its way out of these restraints quite easily, but is not likely to do so while it can detect your immediate presence.

With the others, if you have caught them under a jam-jar, slide a piece of card under and turn the jar up the other way with the animal inside. Loosely fill the jar with shredded paper and either replace the lid, punctured with air holes, or tie a piece of porous material over the top.

Initial Care

In keeping with what we said earlier, the rat will now be left out of consideration, as will the house mouse, although the latter *could* be kept in the manner described hereafter, being of a similar size to the rest of the group.

A 'chew-proof' container is required as a temporary residence, such as an aquarium (without the water of course) or, failing anything else, a biscuit tin. A smaller box in one corner filled with hay will be appreciated by most. This inner box can be of cardboard as it doesn't matter so much if it gets chewed. For a mole, half fill the aquarium or box with soil, and don't bother to provide the inner house since it will not be appreciated.

If using an aquarium with sides of 18in. (45cm) or more, it should not be necessary to provide a cover. With any container less than this height, cover the top as several of the group are quite good at jumping. Whatever is used for the cover must, of course, have air holes, but these must be very tiny as some of these creatures can squeeze through amazingly small spaces. A piece of perforated zinc such as that used for meat safes is ideal for a cover, providing plenty of air through holes much too small for any escape. If using a biscuit tin, the ordinary tin lid can form the cover with plenty of punctures made with a nail. Keep the aquarium/box in a fairly warm room unless the 'client' should be a dormouse which has been scratched out from hibernation (which could be any time between October and April). In this case, place the box in a cool spot with a supply of food (nuts of any kind) as the occupant may wake up from time to time and need a feed. Incidentally, when the dormouse is in hibernation, or even in normal sleep, it appears to be dead and can be moved around quite a bit without waking.

Food
Moles eat earthworms mainly, and in considerable numbers. They will accept a little tinned dog meat from time to time, simply left on the surface of the soil. In common with most of this group, the mole must eat frequently – at least every four hours day and night – in order to survive, so food must be available at all times.

Shrews eat mainly insects. They are partial to woodlice and snails but will also accept small portions of any kind of meat including the tinned varieties.

Nuts are the main diet of a dormouse, but it will also accept grain and chick pellets. The nuts can be left in their shells which the dormouse will make short work of.

Voles eat both insects and a wide variety of vegetable matter. They can be offered tinned dog meat, insectivorous bird food, grain, cereals, apple, berries, vegetables (both root and leaf), and chick pellets.

Apart from the house mouse, there are three other mice in the group, namely the long-tailed field mouse (or wood mouse), the yellow-necked mouse, and the beautiful little harvest mouse, which, with a maximum weight of only about $\frac{1}{4}$oz or 9g, can easily sit on an ear of corn without bending the stem. The harvest mouse eats mainly grain, while the others will accept as wide a variety as the voles as well as clover and dandelion (leaves and flower buds), acorns, various plant bulbs – indeed most things vegetable.

Water must be provided although some drink very little, depending on the moisture content of the food being offered.

Force-feeding
Not a very practical proposition.

Symptoms, Diagnosis and Treatment
Injuries. Rarely, if ever, will a member of this group be found

injured, for the injuries are either fatal or the animal will take itself and its injuries off as fast as possible.

Diseases and Poisoning. Not infrequently, some species – usually rats and mice – may be found poisoned: semi-comatose, lethargic, hunched-up with dishevelled coat. The poison most frequently used today is Warfarin which prevents blood from clotting, causing internal bleeding, and the animal takes a day or so to die.

Strychnine, the poison normally used to kill moles, is cruel, and in fact its use on all animals except moles is forbidden. Because the baited earthworms are put down its tunnel, the horrible symptoms of periodic contraction of the muscles until it dies from asphyxia are not seen.

Voles, harvest mice and shrews may be poisoned by accident with mercury-treated grain used in planting, or by agricultural pesticides, but one never sees a sick animal.

It is rare to come across a diseased mammal from this group, but then one does not often see a healthy one either in the garden or countryside. But, as with all the other wild creatures, disease is a hazard to which many succumb. Rats get a type of typhoid with the general name of salmonella and some types are infectious to man. They are also susceptible to infectious anaemia and to leptospirosis which can affect dogs as well as man. Brucellosis, too, has infected rats as have a number of other diseases. Perhaps their susceptibility to so many diseases explains why they are often used as experimental animals.

Mice are almost as vulnerable, and the spread of disease is enhanced by numbers living close together. Less is known about voles and shrews, though they seem to be susceptible to fewer diseases. Moles have apparently not attracted the attention of the scientists researching disease, for there are few reports in the literature.

As may be expected all small mammals are susceptible to both ecto- and endo-parasites (external and internal). Ticks, mites, fleas and lice all infect this group of small mammals quite commonly. It will be remembered that bubonic plague – the 'black death' which killed millions in Europe during the lifetime of Newton – was spread by fleas to both rats and human beings.

If ectoparasites did not spread disease they would be no more than a nuisance to the host. But fleas are responsible for spreading several diseases including a tapeworm that is common in mice, with the flea acting as its intermediate host. For this reason, some rescuers may wish to dust the animal with a proprietary powder to get rid of them. They are not, however, dangerous to human beings. Ticks are much more difficult to deal with and, fortunately, they do little harm. Their mouth parts are so embedded in the skin of their host that pulling on the body will tear the tick apart leaving the mouth parts in the skin where they sometimes cause irritation and suppuration. A drop of ether or chloroform onto the tick will make it let go and drop off. Alcohol may work too.

General Care

The animal should be housed and cared for as outlined in *Initial Care* until ready for release. There is no advantage to be gained from putting it out of doors, and such a course may well prove detrimental unless placed well in the shade.

Release

In the case of a water shrew or water vole, take the animal to the vicinity of a stream for release. For the rest, simply place the sleeping box under a hedge away from a road. In the case of a dormouse which you have been wintering, make sure the animal is fully awake. You can judge this by the amount of food consumed during the night before release. Although some of the group can be seen during the day, it is best to effect a release just before dark.

Orphans

We have never reared the orphans of any of this group and it is most unlikely you will ever be called upon to do so – which is just as well since we would not rate your chances of success very highly.

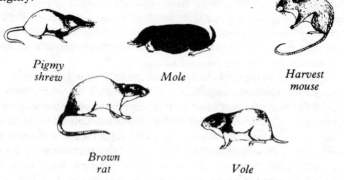

Pigmy shrew

Mole

Harvest mouse

Brown rat

Vole

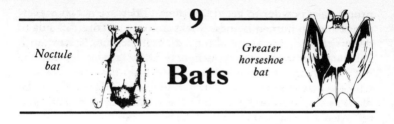

Noctule bat

Greater horseshoe bat

9

Bats

In a contest to find the animal which makes people cringe most, the bat must surely rate very high – certainly in the first three alongside snakes and spiders. Bram Stoker and authors of that ilk bear much of the blame with their tales of vampires, but it must be admitted that the bats themselves do ·not present a very attractive appearance to the average human eye which is, of course, no fault of theirs. Another factor which doesn't help their popularity is their association in most people's minds with belfrys and churchyards, though they can be found in a wide variety of locations. We recently came across a colony living in the roof space of a new council house on a large estate, much to the horror of the tenant who thought it a reflection on her household cleanliness, like having cockroaches in the kitchen (which, incidentally, is also erroneous, see Chapter 22).

Although the vast majority of people have never seen a bat close up – the usual view is of shadowy forms flitting about in the twilight as they catch their evening meal – most people can identify one, although they would probably have no idea which of the native species it might be. The little pipistrelle is by far the most common, and should you stand quite still and silent, will be quite curious about you, and fly quite close, sometimes within inches of your face but never touching you. Others include the great bat or noctule, long eared, whiskered and natterer's bat and the remainder are uncommon.

In flight, a bat makes the average bird look a rank amateur with its incomparable skill and manoeuvrability. They stop, turn at right angles in mid-air, change direction in seemingly impossible ways, and of course they have the added refinement of built-in echo location systems which virtually eliminate the danger of collisions with any obstacle. (Thus you can disabuse yourself of the ridiculous notion that a bat might entangle itself in your hair.) We recently heard a story of a rare collision, but as it was with a fishing line at twilight, the bat can't really be blamed! The person concerned – a girl with long hair – was rather surprised after her inexpert cast to feel tugging in the sky rather than in the river, and to find she'd hooked a bat instead of a plump salmon. She wound the line in, the bat hung confidently from her finger while she gently detached the hook from the wing membrane, and then it flew off happily into the air. A variation on the one that got away!

Of the fifteen species recorded in the UK, the largest is only about 3½in. (9cm) long and even this 'monster' is very rare. An average of the large ones is about 2½–3in. (6.75–7.5cm), and it can do no harm to reiterate that they are all completely inoffensive creatures, which will harm neither man nor his property, even if they *are* squatting in the roof space. Indeed, the greater horseshoe bat and the mouse-eared bat are protected by law (see *Wildlife and the Law*, Appendix A).

Having really no enemies, one would expect them to be very numerous except that they only give birth to one infant each year. The baby is hairless and helpless but it can grab hold of and cling onto its mother who carries it about when she flies out feeding. After a time, however, it gets too big and she will leave it 'hanging about' while she goes out, and will suckle it when she gets back. By the time the baby is seven weeks old, it can fly itself.

All British bat species hibernate between October and April although they may fly out to feed during warm spells in the wintertime if the temperature rises above 7°C (46°F). It is essential for their survival that they hibernate in clusters, for it is their combined body heat which keeps them alive (a solitary bat would just not survive because the temperature would fall below the critical level). They choose caves and lofts with very particular climatic conditions: there must be ventilation but no through draughts, and the moisture content must not be too low.

Possible Handling Hazards

Some species are quite amenable to being handled and do not seem to bother at all, while others will bite and some can draw blood. We hasten to add, before the mention of blood reconjures thoughts of vampires, that they will only bite when you catch hold of them – they will not attack, and they will not lap up the blood their bite might cause!

Approach and Capture

It is quite simple to catch perfectly fit bats, should it be necessary for purposes of relocation (see *General Care*). If you can manage to get into their roosting place, they can just be picked off their perch.

Some bats have difficulty in getting into the air when grounded and require only a lift onto a ledge or tree branch.

Transportation

A dark box is of the essence should you need to transport bats. A cardboard one will be quite adequate, and in it you should firmly wedge a piece of rough timber to which the bats can cling in their normal upside-down posture. They will be much more at ease if offered this simple facility than if just left to crawl about on the bottom of the box.

Initial Care

Bats seldom become genuine casualties and on the comparatively rare occasions we cared for a bat – never for more than one or two days – we have kept it in a box as above with a suitable piece of timber to cling to.

Food

Dried flies (obtainable from pet shops) dampened in a little water appear to be acceptable but again, we cannot claim any great experience on which to base a sound judgement. They have certainly been eaten by one or two of the bats we have kept. A little tinned dog meat could be tried, too, should a bat have to be kept for some time.

Symptoms, Diagnosis and Treatment

The only injury we have ever come across in bats is a torn wing membrane and even this is rather rare because of the animal's great flying skill. A torn membrane can be sutured using fine nylon thread, provided the tear is not too great. The skin or membrane between the elongated fingers is well supplied with blood and if the edges are brought together accurately, it should heal fairly well.

No doubt British bats get diseases and are parasitized, but we have no experience of this. No-one has ever brought a bat to us for treatment other than for a torn membrane.

General Care

We are sorry to offer so little information in the foregoing sections on the care of bats in captivity, but there is little point in airing knowledge which you don't possess. Since we have nothing to add regarding general care in captivity, we thought a few notes on helping to care for bats in the wild might not come amiss.

There are three types of roost used by bats in this country – buildings, hollow trees, and caves. Caves are only used in the winter during hibernation and of the other two, buildings are used more extensively, but only those parts that are not being used by human residents – roof spaces, wall cavities, or indeed anywhere which offers good shelter but is reasonably 'private'.

It is fair to say that they are good neighbours. They do not make a lot of noise (at least not that you can hear), do not make nests or damage the building in any way, their droppings are dry and very nearly odourless and do not have any of the corrosive qualities of bird droppings. They are clean and prefer to live in a clean environment and, last but not least, they are night-shift workers so they don't bother you at all during the day. In fact all they do is very strictly mind their own business which in no way intrudes on that of the other residents of the building. They are so unobtrusive that very often people are quite unaware they are on the premises.

Having said all that, all the begging, pleading and cajoling you can muster will not persuade some people who will flatly refuse to have bats in their house. On one occasion a chap turned up with a box containing thirty-seven long-eared bats which he'd been obliged to remove from his roof space. His wife had left the house immediately she learned they were there and refused to enter again until the poor old bats were forcibly ejected! Such extreme cases are rare, fortunately, since removal in this manner is not a good idea. Most people who want to get rid of bats are prepared to 'serve notice to quit' and allow a reasonable time for the eviction to be executed. The procedure recommended by the Royal Society for Nature Conservation is the best one to follow, and we quote from their interesting leaflet, *Focus on Bats.*

'The whereabouts of exit holes and the approximate number of bats present should be ascertained by watching on two consecutive evenings from sunset to darkness. During the next day, little-used holes should be sealed with appropriate materials, leaving the main exit open. The same evening, bats should be counted again whilst they are emerging to forage and when all appear to have left, rags should be pushed firmly into the hole preventing their return. Early the following evening, the rags should be removed so as to allow any further bats to escape before finally filling the hole.

'If this method is adopted, *two important precautions* must be taken to ensure that dead rotting bodies are not left in the building causing smell and damage. First, no action be taken between mid-June and about the 20th of August because young bats remain in the roof when mother leaves to feed. Secondly, avoid action during cold weather because none or only a few bats will emerge to feed each evening.'

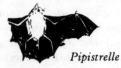

Pipistrelle

Long-eared bat

10

Hedgehogs

No-one could possibly mistake a hedgehog for anything else, and the smallest child can usually give a fair description of its distinctive appearance, without knowing anything else about it or ever having seen one. Its coat of spines is a feature shared by no other indigenous mammal, and everyone seems to have a 'soft spot' for this harmless and wholly admirable little animal. If one should appear in the garden, who can resist rushing in to prepare some extra nourishment for the visitor, and who would not be delighted if a hedgehog should honour them by taking up residence in the vicinity?

The hedgehog is very useful to man, for it eats many garden pests. However, there are old country superstitions that hedgehogs will take the eggs of game birds, even killing a sitting bird, and that they will suck milk from cows. Whilst it is true that the hedgehog may occasionally take an abandoned egg, a moment's reflection will show how ridiculous it is to suggest that hedgehogs can suck milk from cows. Their mouths are far too small to contain the teat of the cow for a start, and their sharp teeth would soon have the cow on its feet and out of reach. They may be seen *near* resting cows, but this is probably due to the cow's heat encouraging the insects which are the hedgehog's main food. If a hedgehog is presented with a hen's egg, it finds it impossible to eat, for it cannot break through the shell; its mouth is simply not big enough.

Hedgehogs lay down fat during the summer to supply all their bodily needs for the winter hibernation. They lay down two types of fat: the normal white fat with each cell containing one large globule; and also brown fat where each cell contains several fat globules and tiny microscopic structures called mitochondria. It is these that can burn up fat to produce heat, about twenty times faster than white fat. This mechanism is activated by a drop in external temperature, and therefore the colder it gets the more heat brown fat produces. At the same time the animal's metabolism (all its bodily functions) slows down, its temperature falls, its heart rate slows and its breathing can hardly be detected.

This means that the amount of energy needed to keep the animal alive is very much reduced.

Possible Handling Hazards

There is little danger of being bitten by a hedgehog but the spines are very sharp and a prick will leave a lingering tingle, similar to being stung by a nettle. When threatened, the hedgehog will roll itself into a ball, presenting the spines in virtually every direction and deterring most adversaries.

Approach and Capture

A hedgehog which is still mobile can move surprisingly quickly, but is not too difficult to overtake. Avoid letting it get under a hedge or indeed under anything else where it will prove most difficult to extricate. An adult is quite difficult to pick up when rolled in a ball. As already indicated, the spines are very sharp indeed and the pressure of grip which needs to be exerted in order to lift the animal will cause painful pricks to bare hands. Anything which can be pierced by a needle can equally be pierced by a hedgehog spine so a pair of thin gloves may afford no protection although a leather pair will probably solve the problem. If no suitable gloves are available, lay out a handkerchief and roll the animal onto it, picking it up easily by the four handkerchief corners in sling fashion. If your handkerchief isn't large enough – most ladies' handkerchiefs aren't, and even a man's might be rather small to span a large boar hedgehog – a newspaper will serve the same purpose.

Transportation

Any kind of container or no container at all will be quite in order. Your patient is unlikely to make much of a fuss during the journey and may well remain rolled up for the whole of it. There is no problem even if it does decide to have a walk about, as it isn't likely to make a sudden leap out of the window, nor will it attempt to savage your ankle!

Initial Care

It's important to bear in mind that the hedgehog is a hibernating species and if your patient has been found between October and March (or even April), it may well have accidentally or intentionally been dug out from its winter nest and may still be sound asleep. It is by no means an unusual occurrence for a blissfully slumbering hedgehog to be raked out from its snug winter quarters under a pile of dead leaves by a keen gardener doing a bit of tidying up, and quite unaware of the animal's presence. A dog, ambling about seeking diversion, may notice an interesting odour emanating from the dead leaf pile and dig out the poor old hedgehog just from curiosity.

It is quite difficult to detect signs of life in a hibernating animal and poking it just to see if it moves is not recommended. If there is reason to suspect the animal may merely be in hibernation (and the time of year is the obvious guide to this), it should be placed in a box containing hay, straw or dry dead leaves and the box deposited somewhere weatherproof, but unheated, and with an easy means of exit. The deep sleep may have been disturbed and the hedgehog may wake up and wish to take itself off elsewhere. Some sleep only intermittently during part of the hibernation, in any case, and must be able to get out from wherever you have placed the box.

It may seem the most obvious thing to do, but it is *not* a good idea to simply put the animal back under the leaves where it was found. The disturbance will have destroyed the lining of the hibernaculum (nest) which was carefully prepared prior to retirement, besides which, if it was the dog that did the original excavation, it will undoubtedly repeat the performance at the first opportunity! (But, of course, if you haven't disturbed its nest *too* much, carefully cover it up and leave it where it is.)

For a *bona fide* casualty, a cardboard box filled as above will make an ideal temporary residence, and if it can be placed in a room from which there is no escape, the box can be placed on its side, allowing the patient to come out at night if it so wishes (assuming it is mobile). When considering where to house your patient, bear in mind that hedgehogs usually carry fleas in large numbers (see *Symptoms, Diagnosis and Treatment*).

It may be desirable in certain circumstances to provide additional heat but it is not usually necessary. The hedgehog does its normal sleeping during the warmest part of each twenty-four-hour cycle.

Food

Nourishment should be provided from the start, putting the food out in the evening ready for the patient's awakening. Hedgehogs are very easy to cater for. Tinned dog or cat meat and a dish of water will be quite acceptable and quite sufficient, although a dish of bread and milk will be appreciated. Make sure the dishes are low enough for the animal to be able to reach in comfortably and don't be stingy with the meat. A hedgehog will eat rather more than you would expect from its size. Other things, such as a broken raw egg, can be offered. Indeed a hedgehog will have a go at virtually anything you would eat yourself – as well as a number of other things you wouldn't care to sample – but if it is getting a dish of dog or cat meat, there will be no complaint and the patient will thrive.

Force-feeding

A hedgehog will normally feed readily in captivity and if it fails to do so, there is likely to be something very seriously wrong which precludes it doing so (a broken jaw, for example). Force-feeding is not very satisfactory since an injury which prevents this particular species from eating is likely to be one which is not amenable to treatment. There is also the actual physical problem of trying to feed an animal which curls up into a ball with the mouth in the centre of the ball! But, as with all animals, hedgehogs have a degree of individuality, and it is not too difficult to gain the confidence of some, so that they do not keep curling up every time you approach. If your patient is one of these, and you think it necessary, warm milk with a pinch of glucose added can be trickled into the mouth in the manner described later for orphans.

Symptoms, Diagnosis and Treatment

Injuries. By far the most common injury is caused on the road by motor cars, for the animal seems to have a propensity to wander across roads, perhaps to feed on insects killed by cars, and can't get out of the way quickly enough. Thousands are slaughtered on the roads every year. It seems somewhat ironic that here is an animal useful about the garden, eating up slugs and sundry pests, which doesn't do us any harm at all, is almost universally liked, and yet we have still managed to devise a means (albeit unintentional) of killing it.

A fox or a badger, hard pressed for a meal, may occasionally tackle a hedgehog, but in general its only real enemy is the motor car.

In the majority of cases the animal is killed, or is so severely injured that it must be put to sleep. Occasionally, however, the injuries may be slight enough to warrant treatment and the main problem is getting the patient to unroll so that a proper examination can be made. Opening by force is liable to cause further injury. Placing the animal in a shallow pool of water or puffing some tobacco smoke onto it will usually do the trick. One person must hold it open by placing one hand across its body immediately behind the forelegs and the other just in front of the rear legs while a second person attends to the injury. A fracture in the lower part of the leg is easily diagnosed and can be splinted, but a fracture higher up is a job for a veterinary surgeon.

However, if the animal is kept and nursed as recommended in *Initial Care* and *General Care*, healing will probably take place of its own accord. Even if the animal has a slight limp, it will not affect its ability to feed nor very much alter its speed of escape.

Diseases. The hedgehog is susceptible to salmonella, pseudo-tuberculosis and leptospira (a group of diseases that affects the liver and kidneys). It is most unlikely that a member of the public will find a sick hedgehog, but if they do they should take it immediately to a veterinary surgeon.

Hedgehogs are sometimes parasitized by ticks, usually ixodes hexagonus. It is most unlikely that this parasite will attach itself to a human being and it certainly will not remain there. They should not be pulled off as this breaks off the sucking parts which remain buried in the skin and may suppurate. Fleas are regularly found in hedgehogs for they can be more easily seen than on thick-furred animals. They will rarely parasitize humans. It is wiser not to attempt to deinfest hedgehogs. Wild animals have become adapted, on the whole, to parasites.

General Care
If a period of convalescence should be thought necessary prior to release, do not think you can contain the animal with a simple wire fence. Hedgehogs are excellent climbers and will easily scale any wire fence or ivy-clad wall, and even trees from time to time. Any enclosure for a hedgehog must, therefore, either have completely smooth walls – corrugated iron or asbestos, for example. If it must be made with any kind of wire mesh, the top too must be covered like an aviary, or the boundary fence must have an overhang (see Fig. 14). It is also advisable to take the boundary fencing material at least a few inches underground. Hedgehogs don't dig much, but will worry away at the smallest gap under a fence until it is large enough to crawl through.

Some cover must be provided within the enclosure where the animal can sleep during the day. In the absence of anything natural, a simple wooden box on its side and filled with bedding, as already described, will be quite satisfactory. In very hot weather, try to provide some additional shade for the box and point the open end away from the sun.

Release
Providing the plants and ground aren't sprayed all over with pesticides and strewn with slug pellets, and you're not on a main road, you couldn't do better for yourself *and* the hedgehog than to release it into your own garden. If it decides to stay around –

and you may influence the decision by a little judicious bribery in the shape of a dish of milk and a light snack each night – you will have a valuable gardening assistant on whose menu slugs and snails come high in preference.

If you don't have a satisfactory situation for a release on home ground, take the hedgehog to any reasonably quiet spot away from main roads and pop it under a hedge just after dark when it is waking up and will have the whole night to sort itself out.

Orphans

This is one species where a good many genuine orphans do occur owing to the very heavy death toll on the roads. The first indication of infants in distress will usually be a high pitched peeping sound, more reminiscent of a bird than a mammal, emanating from under a hedge or a well-grown shrub. This sound can be taken as a clear indication that the sow has failed to return to the nest after a foraging expedition the previous night, or possibly even the night before that. Tracing the sound to its source, the infants may be found clear of the nest and crawling about in search of their mother, even when still blind, or they may be found still in the nest but very cold. On one occasion, tracing the characteristic peeping to the nest, one of us found a badly injured dead sow with the tiny, uncomprehending infants still trying to gain warmth and nourishment from her. Who knows just how far and in what pain she had struggled heroically to get back to her family.

When first born, the youngsters are pink with soft, almost white spines but stronger darker spines begin to appear within two or three days. The eyes begin to open at about two weeks by which time they are the adult colour with spines which can already give quite a prick. They gain the ability to curl up into a ball about two days before their eyes open and are quite efficient at it from this very early age. They are also very quick to learn that although the strange creature handling them isn't mum, it will provide suitable nourishment.

Orphaned hedgehogs will invariably arrive chilled. It is probably this as much as hunger that prompts the distress signal. The first essential, therefore, is to provide warmth of some sort. A wrapped hot water bottle will do the trick in the short term but something of a more constant temperature is needed with a dull-emitter infra-red heater as the favourite. A cardboard box with an open top and one open end should be filled with hay, covering the infants, and the heater suspended over it. A 250 watt heater with reflector, suspended about 18in. (45cm) above *the base of* the box, will give about the right amount of heat. The open end to the box allows for ventilation and also allows the youngsters to crawl away if a steep rise in the ambient temperature should heat the box too much.

Use ordinary cow's milk mixed with 50 per cent water and a pinch of glucose to each feed. Make the mixture warm by using warm water and mix a fresh lot each time.

If starting from the new-born (pink) stage, feed two hourly throughout the day, fitting in eight or nine feeds – starting at 7 am and finishing at 11 pm. If you do this, there is no need to go on through the night too. Allow 1 teaspoon (5ml) per feed for each youngster although they will probably only manage about half a teaspoon (3ml) at first. They will feed best lying on their backs. We always use a 5ml plastic syringe for the job. The youngsters will find this a bit awkward to cope with at first and are likely to dribble quite a lot – hence the 5ml size when only about 3ml are likely to be actually swallowed. The main advantage of a syringe is that the flow can easily be controlled and also the quantity easily measured. The best way to go about it is to sit on a low stool (or on the floor) with a towel over your lap on which to lay the infants in turn, belly upwards with head away from you. Insert the tip of the syringe into the corner of the mouth and the infant will immediately start chewing on it and taking in the mixture at the same time. Press the plunger *very slowly*, stopping whenever the mouth fills up with the mixture, indicating that swallowing has stopped for a moment. As the infant reaches capacity, it will stop swallowing altogether and the mixture will simply dribble out of the sides of the mouth.

Continue with this same number of feeds for the first week, at the end of which each youngster should be taking the full teaspoon (5ml). The number of feeds can then be reduced to six and a little more offered at each feed. After another week the eyes should be opening and the youngsters will start to move around, at which stage a low dish with some tinned dog or cat meat with some diluted milk poured over it should be placed near at hand.

The youngsters won't take long to get the idea of feeding although their early efforts are likely to prove very messy indeed as they will insist on wading into the centre of the dish, eating and lapping as they go. Hand feeding should continue until they are well established at feeding themselves, gradually reducing the frequency of feeds as they take more solid food. They should be feeding well by four to five weeks and hand feeding can then cease.

By the fifth week, they should also no longer need a heater. In fact it may be possible to cut this off after about three weeks, but this will depend a good deal on the ambient temperature. Some summers are a great deal warmer than others. A good idea is to place another box similarly furnished but away from the heater. As the original becomes too warm for comfort, you may find the infants move to the other, in which case you can turn off the heater. But do be ready to turn it on again at any sharp decline in temperature.

Once they have dispensed with the heater and are feeding themselves entirely, a move outside can be made, with much the same set-up as for adult casualties. Bear in mind, though, that the youngsters will be able to get out of much smaller holes than adults.

We recommend about eight weeks for complete release by which time they should be able to cope with life perfectly well. But there is one proviso. Second litters can be born as late in the year as September and if you should have such a litter, it may be better (for them) to consider letting them hibernate within the enclosure. They need to put on a good deal of fat to survive the winter and in the wild, many second-litter youngsters do not make it. If you provide plenty of accommodation within the enclosure and continue to feed them until they retire, they will have a much better chance of appearing again in the spring. We can well do with a few more saved to help make up the losses on the roads.

If you are 'wintering them over', put out a bit of food on mild nights (if any!) just in case any of the sleepers should emerge and go looking for something to eat and/or drink. Make the final release as soon as your charges are awake, which may be in March but is more likely in April. Alternatively, they can be kept indoors in warm quarters where they will continue to feed throughout the winter.

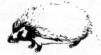

Hedgehog

11

Hares and Rabbits

The rabbit is probably the most familiar of all wild mammals and, apart from the agricultural community which places it rather low in the popularity stakes, is familiar to and loved by most of us – reared as we are on a diet of endearing characters such as Peter Rabbit and that most debonair cartoon personality, Bugs Bunny, delightful little Easter bunnies decorating shop windows and, in recent years, the splendid cast of Richard Adams' *Watership Down*. Rabbits have also been kept as domestic pets for a long time, and are now to be found in all shapes and sizes, so people generally feel closer to the rabbit than to other wild mammals.

Many look upon the wild population too as 'pets' and wouldn't hesitate to pick one up. Even its severest critics could not deny its winsome appearance with those outsize ears and back feet, that perky expression and hopping gait, brought up at the rear with that little white powderpuff of a tail. There is really little wonder it has been anthropomorphized out of all recognition.

There are two types of hare. The brown hare can be found in most parts of the country and the blue is found in Scotland and Ireland, with small pockets in the North of England and North Wales. The blue hare is not really blue, more a sort of browny-grey, and in winter its coat becomes partially white.

There is much interesting fact and folk-lore about hares. For instance, they are reputed to be able to run faster up a hill than down and to purposely lead any pursuer up a hill, should there be one in the vicinity, where they can demonstrate their superiority. The antics of the 'mad March hare' are a joy to watch should you ever chance to view the spectacle. They aren't really mad of course – the leaping about and sparring with each other only *look* mad to us. It is mating behaviour and doubtless very serious to the hares!

Although hares and rabbits belong to the same family of animals and look very much alike, from the point of view of caring for them in captivity, there is one very significant difference (see *Orphans*). There are many other physical differences between hares and rabbits but the easiest one to remember is that all hares have black tips to the ears (even the blue in its winter coat) and rabbits do not.

Possible Handling Hazards

Many people unhesitatingly pick up a hare or rabbit, never dreaming that there could be any danger from 'a bunny'. In the majority of cases this is right, but both the rabbit and the hare can, and sometimes do, bite, and the bite can be quite severe. They frequently cause painful scratches with the hind feet. Although this is by accident in an attempt to escape rather than by design, it doesn't lessen the pain!

Approach and Capture

If one of this group is still mobile, your chances of catching it are virtually nil. It is only when the injury is incapacitating that there is any chance of approaching the animal. There is an old theory, though, that you can come right up to a perfectly fit hare by walking around it in decreasing circles, and we tested it once on a hare which was sitting virtually in the middle of a three-acre meadow. Starting with a very wide circle, the approach was made walking slowly but quite steadily and not looking at the animal directly until no more than 12 feet (3.5 metres) separated the walker from the 'subject'. At that point, the hare decided it had seen enough of this idiot wandering around in circles and bolted, but proving, however, that there was some truth in the theory.

On being approached, an injured animal will frequently give a piercing scream of sheer terror which can be a bit unnerving if you haven't heard it before. Doing all the handling slowly and gently with no sudden movements will do much to calm this terror.

It is quite in order for one hand to hold the ears – indeed it is the best way to avoid being bitten – but the other hand *must* support the weight of the body when lifting. A rabbit or hare should never be lifted by the ears alone. Place the supporting hand so that you avoid scratches to the forearm from the hind feet. Under the rump is the best position.

Transportation

A member of this group will appreciate being in the dark, and a stout cardboard box will serve for a short journey. Although a fit hare or rabbit could very easily demolish such a container, one that is injured is more likely to be grateful for the seclusion. Don't forget to provide a few air holes. For longer journeys and those where an eye cannot be kept on the container during the trip, a wicker cat basket is ideal. Cover it with a coat or something to make it darker inside but be sure ample air can get in.

Initial Care

The animal will most appreciate being left alone in a quiet place with a soft bed of hay or straw to recover from the initial trauma of the injury, and the capture and handling. Place a handful of grass, clover, and/or dandelion within reach and also a shallow bowl of water, and leave the patient overnight unless there is some wound requiring immediate attention. There should normally be no need to provide artificial heat for an adult member of this group and it may even be detrimental to do so.

Food

Hares and rabbits are easy to cater for, especially during the summer months. Give them grass, clover, dandelion, coltsfoot, carrot and turnip tops, cabbage, grain, cereals or apple, and if hay is provided for bedding, they are also likely to consume some of this.

Water should always be available. Serve it in the heaviest available bowl you have as members of this group always seem curious to see what is under a bowl, and are likely to turn it over.

It is natural and necessary for hares and rabbits to eat some of their own faeces as this is part of the digestive process.

Force-feeding

Not recommended. If your patient cannot feed itself, its chances of survival are very small and it is unlikely to be helped by attempted force-feeding.

Symptoms, Diagnosis and Treatment

Injuries. Road accidents are the usual causes of injury to rabbits and more often than not one or more legs are broken. If the injuries are extensive it may be kinder to put the animal to sleep. Occasionally one may be found entangled in a snare, and again if a limb is badly damaged, or there is a great loss of skin, it may be a kindness to put the animal to sleep. Sometimes a young rabbit may be carried home by a dog or a cat, or during a country walk you may surprise a stoat or a weasel that has just caught a young rabbit. In these cases the animal is often so shocked that there is little chance of recovery, but this is not always the case.

The minor wounds can be treated at home in the usual way, but major lacerations and broken legs are best taken to the veterinary surgeon.

Diseases. Rabbits and hares are susceptible, like most animals, to a variety of diseases, but the one most commonly found by the British public is myxomatosis. From time to time a hare has been found with this disease, but it is the rabbit that is most often discovered, usually in an appalling state.

In the 1930s it was estimated that there were thirty million rabbits in Britain and in the 1950s this had risen to between sixty and one hundred million. Almost two rabbits for every man, woman and child in the country. The numbers had been increasing in France, too, and in the early 50s, a French farmer imported the myxomatosis virus from Australia where it had been used to reduce vast populations of rabbits. He infected two rabbits and released them on his estate. It began to spread and soon got out of control. A British farmer noticed the great reduction in rabbit populations that had been caused by this disease and introduced it into Britain in 1953.

The virus is spread on the whole by the rabbit flea, which flourishes in the intimacy of the rabbit burrows, and it is interesting that many rabbits now seem to be living above ground in some areas. In the open air, there is less likelihood of the flea jumping from rabbit to rabbit. The symptoms of myxomatosis are swelling of the eyelids and the base of the ears which eventually prevents the animal from seeing and hearing. It also causes diarrhoea, debility and depression, so that the animal sits around in a miserable state and is an easy prey for its predators. There is no treatment, and because over 90 per cent eventually die it is kinder to put the animal to sleep immediately.

Rabbits are also affected by parasites, both coccidiosis and worms, but are rarely found in the diseased state, the public is unlikely to have to diagnose or treat these conditions.

General Care

Any outdoor enclosure should have the added refinement of wire netting on the base otherwise your patient is very likely to indulge in a bit of excavation during the night. Do not be lulled into thinking that because your patient is a hare and hares do not burrow in the wild, it will not attempt to dig its way out, otherwise you may well awaken to an empty pen! Incidentally, there are now many rabbits too which do not burrow in the wild. This appears to date from the time of the introduction of myxomatosis in the 1950s (see *Symptoms, Diagnosis and Treatment*) when many rabbits took to a life on the surface.

The outside pen need not be very tall and the easiest type to construct is one of triangular shape (on the end) with a simple covered section at one end and the rest covered in wire netting (see Fig. 9). 2in. (5cm) mesh is best for the base, allowing grass to poke through, and the pen can be moved to a new position each day. This assumes you have an area of grass, but if you haven't the animal should still be moved out of doors as soon as possible, even if the pen has to be placed on concrete.

If the pen is on grass, there is no need to provide anything more elaborate by way of a house than the simple shelter illustrated. Bear in mind that although they look like them, these are *not* domestic pets (which require rather more cosseting for a happy life).

Release

Do not keep the animal penned up longer than absolutely necessary. As soon as it is reasonably fit and able to move at speed, let it out to take its chance, and its best chance will be as far away as possible from arable farmland.

Orphans

It is with the young that the major difference between hares and rabbits lies and it is quite a startling difference. Baby rabbits are born blind, deaf, virtually bald, and quite incapable of movement, whereas baby hares (leverets) are born fully developed with eyes open and capable of hopping about virtually from birth. Leverets are very near indeed to the story-book images of the 'Easter bunny'.

When dealing with young, it must be remembered that a new-born leveret resembles a rabbit which is nearly three weeks old and not far from being able to exist independently (which both can do at about four weeks). Consequently the leveret appears to need bottle-feeding much longer than the rabbit. For bottle-feeding use a half milk, half water mixture with an added pinch of glucose. Five or six feeds a day is adequate and feeding during the night is not necessary. Each youngster will take anything from $\frac{1}{5}-\frac{1}{3}$oz (6–10 ml) per feed. Watch for the mouth filling up and *remaining* full which is an indication that the youngster has had enough. A plastic syringe is the best feeding bottle.

By about the middle of the third week, baby rabbits will be starting to nibble food, leverets sometimes earlier, but both should still be bottle fed, reducing the number of feeds as the intake of solids increases, and both should be quite finished and on a completely adult diet by the end of the fourth week. It will do no harm to put down a dish of milk for them to drink themselves for a further week.

Ideally, the 'nursery' should consist of a long wooden box with solid sides to keep out draughts. The floor can be covered with sawdust, wood shavings or thick newspaper, and at one end make a nest of hay or shredded paper tissues. Provide a bit of warmth around the nest area in the early days, particularly for baby rabbits, but do not make it too hot. Around 20°C (68°F) is adequate. An infra-red dull-emitter is best but an ordinary red electric light bulb as used in electric fires will do. The bedding should be kept dry and this may mean a complete change every day, depending on the number of youngsters in the nest.

Turn off any artificial heat after two weeks and move the youngsters out of doors as soon as possible after they are weaned. The type of pen suggested for adult casualties will suit youngsters equally well but baby rabbits in particular are rather slippery customers and will squeeze through anything their heads will fit. They will quite easily get through 2in. (5cm) mesh netting so 1in. (2.5cm) mesh is advised.

Do not keep the youngsters any longer than is absolutely necessary to ensure complete self-sufficiency and effect release in the manner suggested for adult casualties.

Rabbit

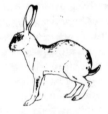

Brown hare

12

Squirrels

Most people would easily identify a squirrel although they are more likely to have encountered the imported grey than the native red. The red favours dense woodland and is nowhere near as cocky and cheeky as its North American counterpart which is quite happy to live in the closest proximity to man. One we were acquainted with persistently climbed into the house through an upstairs toilet window – which it could only reach by negotiating a perilous series of drainpipes and gutters – to sprawl out for a nap on the fluffy cover of the lavatory seat!

In general appearance the species are alike, and the names are accurate in that the red squirrel is red in colour and the grey is grey. But the grey sports a quite noticeable reddish patch on its back, and this occasionally causes confusion. The grey cannot however match the distinctive ear tufts which the red has in winter. It is reasonable to assume, all things considered, that any squirrel encountered in a public place is a grey.

Many people still believe that when the grey squirrel was imported and began to spread, it ousted the red and forced it back to more remote parts. This is not true, as the red was in fact decimated by an epidemic. There have been a number of efforts since, aimed at the total extermination of the grey squirrel (mentioned later), but these have had little or no effect on the total population or indeed the local population in any given area. It could be described as a very successful animal.

Possible Handling Hazards

As with hares and rabbits, appearances can be most deceiving, and a set of teeth like well-honed chisels are concealed behind that jaunty, friendly demeanour which they are not averse to using when circumstances warrant, such as when some well-meaning person is trying to take hold of them. They can inflict a quite substantial injury or injuries which could well need a few stitches.

Approach and Capture

A squirrel, even an injured one which is still mobile, is fast moving and agile, with the added ability of being able to shin rapidly up trees and even rough walls. Short of employing elaborate netting, there is little chance of a successful capture and even with the aid of nets, there is every likelihood the squirrel will still make you look a fool. In approaching one which is apparently incapacitated, it is a good idea to get between the animal and any tree or wall it might still be able to scale, in spite of its injury.

A *very strong* glove, preferably a gauntlet, is recommended for picking up squirrels. Otherwise have the open travelling container very near to hand and pick the squirrel up by the tail, depositing it quickly into the container. It is possible to do this without damage to the animal and with no apparent pain because of the squirrel's very light weight, but the manoeuvre must be completed quickly, before the animal begins to struggle.

Transportation

A healthy squirrel can easily chew its way out of a wooden box but such a container should last the journey home with an injured one. For a journey of any great length, some kind of metal box (a biscuit tin, for instance) would be preferable, remembering of course to puncture plenty of air holes in it. Squirrels are not at all keen on being shut in a completely closed box, so don't keep the animal confined any longer than absolutely necessary.

Initial Care

An indication has already been given of the squirrel's prowess at demolishing timber so do not simply shut it in a room of your house and expect the fixtures and fittings to remain intact, even if the patient appears to be totally incapacitated. Equally, there is not a lot of point in shutting it in a garden shed unless the shed is constructed of brick or concrete block or something equally 'gnaw proof'.

In the early stages, you really cannot do better than an ordinary bird cage. It does not have the claustrophobic effect of a closed box and at the same time it can be partially covered with a cloth to offer a measure of seclusion. Don't cover it with one of your best table cloths or the squirrel is sure to pull it through the bars and tear it to ribbons. An old cloth that you don't want will probably be left alone! Cover the floor of the cage with sawdust for preference although newspaper will do. Provide some food and water then leave the patient alone pending examination.

Food

Nuts rank high in popularity with squirrels. Ordinary peanuts will do nicely, with or without the shells, but not salted. In addition, a wide variety of other things will be accepted and devoured with evident relish. In the Army, when someone eats and apparently enjoys anything and everything placed before him, they say he is 'a good man at the trough'. A squirrel could fairly be described thus as it never turns up its nose at anything. Greens, vegetables, fruit, cereals, chick pellets, even the occasional biscuit and jam or peanut butter sandwich! Nuts should be offered every day with other things on the list as and when available.

Force-feeding

A squirrel, even an injured one, will normally eat quite readily in captivity, so if it doesn't there is something preventing it, and that something will almost certainly be serious enough to warrant the decision to destroy the animal. Force-feeding is not recommended both for this reason and for the hazard to the hands of the feeder. *Squirrel bites are not to be underestimated.*

Symptoms, Diagnosis and Treatment

Injuries. Squirrels, either red or grey, are rarely found injured. Their most common injury is being hit by a car, and this is infrequent. Even more rare is for a young squirrel to be caught by a dog or a cat. The red squirrel is so shy that it is almost never found near human habitat, while the grey squirrel, although forward and cheeky, is very alert and quick in its movements and always seems to escape predators.

Unless the injury is slight it is best to take the animal to a veterinary surgeon for treatment or to be put to sleep.

Diseases and Poisoning. Squirrels are susceptible to diseases, some of which have not yet been diagnosed. In 1960, for example, the outbreak and course of a disease was recorded in a community of red squirrels in Shropshire. It lasted about one week, and the mortality approached 100 per cent. The symptoms started with conjunctivitis, then a nasal discharge, and the lips became swollen and the inside of the mouth sore and ulcerated. By the fifth day there was a throat swelling and soon after the animal became blind, weak and unable to eat, and very quickly died.

This disease, which was a virus disease, is thought to be the one that spread gradually through the separate communities of red squirrels, decimating the English and Welsh populations. One theory postulates that the introduction of the grey squirrel (who seems to be immune) from North America in 1876 brought this disease which affected the red squirrel so badly. Anyway, as the red squirrels disappeared from an area so the greys colonized it.

Squirrels are also susceptible to leptospirosis and can be parasitized by ticks and lice. It is most improbable, however, that a member of the public will ever find a diseased squirrel.

What they may find, however, is a squirrel hunched up and disinclined to move, or perhaps dead or dying. This will occur in or near moorland where poison bait has been laid in a hopper (food trough). Squirrels attack and damage hard-wood trees and Warfarin is often laid to kill them. This drug is an anti-coagulant and the affected animal suffers internal haemorrhages. There is no treatment and the animal should be put to sleep.

General Care

A squirrel could undoubtedly chew a hole in the ordinary lightweight wire netting normally used for garden aviaries as its gnawing abilities, especially through wood, are prodigious. But we have never seen any of our squirrel 'clients' even attempt to bite wire. It's unlikely the squirrels are aware this particular barrier is too strong for them, more likely that chewing wire in order to effect an escape simply has no appeal. The aviary in which we have always housed squirrels is made of 1in. (2.5cm) mesh chain link (apparently no longer available) and this has always proved entirely secure. If an outside pen is to be specially constructed, Twilweld is the material to use. This is a type of strong wire mesh welded at each intersection, which comes in a wide variety of mesh sizes and wire thicknesses. It is much more rigid than ordinary wire netting and also much more durable. A 1in. (2.5cm) mesh with a wire thickness of 16 gauge would be suitable for squirrels and would also 'double' as an aviary for a wide variety of birds.

It is quite safe to house a squirrel in an aviary containing birds of the crow family, pigeons, pheasants, etc., as well as rabbits and guinea pigs. There may be a bit of initial chasing around but little likelihood of harm to either side. It may even be safe to house a squirrel with smaller birds but not having tried this, we cannot recommend it.

It is generally accepted that squirrels will take bird's eggs and even nestlings, but we housed one particular grey squirrel in an aviary where pigeons regularly laid eggs, and the squirrel took no interest in them whatsoever. Nor did it attempt to harm any squeakers (baby pigeons). It even occupied the top compartment of a pigeon cote within the aviary with pigeons and jackdaws occupying the rest!

A small wooden box about a foot square will be readily adopted as a drey (nest) if it is fastened up on the side wire of the pen. It is best to let the squirrel itself do the furnishing. Throw a couple of handfuls of hay on the ground and the squirrel will collect it up and carry it to the drey. Incidentally, they appear to prefer two entrances to their residence and if you only provide one, the squirrel is likely to chew out another one itself.

It is preferable that at least part of the ground area should be grass. The squirrel will not attempt to dig itself out but does like somewhere to bury nuts which it will do by carefully parting the topsoil to both sides while holding the nut in its mouth. The nut will then be placed in the small hole and the topsoil rapidly but carefully patted back in place.

Release

Squirrels do not hibernate but if you have one late in the season, it would be best to keep it until the spring since it will have no 'winter larder' stored away (as above) and should the winter be a hard one, may find difficulty in surviving.

Squirrels are very unpopular with foresters, especially the grey, and there is no doubt they do considerable damage, particularly to very young trees. If and when you are releasing a squirrel try to do so in a piece of old woodland as far away from plantations as possible.

Orphans

The felling of a tree containing a nursery drey may well produce squirrel infants in need of care and rearing. Older babies, not yet adept at the art of climbing, frequently fall out of trees, and these should be left alone as the mother will almost certainly be along to attend to them.

Baby squirrels adapt quite readily to a human foster parent, even from their very early days when they are blind and naked.

The first essential is the provision of a warm, snug artificial drey – a high-sided cardboard or wooden box which will keep out the draughts, or even a large plastic plantpot. You will ultimately want to place the drey-substitute inside a cage – when the babies start to move around – so bear this in mind when you choose the size of your drey. For bedding, put in plenty of paper tissues or, better still, a generous amount of the new type of pet bedding, made of finely shredded paper, sold by most pet shops. Artificial heat should be provided to keep the drey at about 25 C (86 F) constant. The airing cupboard may provide the right spot providing it is well ventilated and doesn't get too hot.

Initial feeding should be on the same mixture and at the same rate as for baby rabbits (Chapter 11, page 101), but will need to be continued for at least five weeks, which is about two weeks after the eyes open, and thereafter until they can feed themselves properly at about eight weeks. About a week after the eyes open is the time to start offering a little more solid food. As you lift each one out for a feed, have a shallow dish of bread and diluted warm milk handy and offer it *before* giving the 'bottle'. At first there will be little response but, if the youngsters have been brought in very young and have consequently been hand fed for quite some time, they will associate being lifted out of the drey with having food. If this is withheld for a few moments and the youngster's mouth is steered in the direction of the dish, it will quite soon get the idea. The bottle feeding must continue as indicated above.

As soon as the youngsters show interest in coming out of the drey of their own accord, it is time to move them (and the drey) into a cage but still indoors. There should, by this time, be no need to continue the artificial heating, but do keep the cage up off the floor in case of draughts. Obviously the larger the cage the better and a close-meshed parrot cage is ideal. Put at least one piece of tree branch in for climbing practice.

Continue to provide the bread and milk which was their first introduction to solid food but begin to introduce other things. Pieces of apple and chick pellets are good starters, as well as nuts, of course, but these should be shelled first. A dish of water should also be provided and should remain at all times.

When they are feeding themselves entirely they can be moved out of doors at which time they can be provided with conditions similar to those for adult casualties. Put some bedding in the sleeping box for them, though, as they won't quite have the knack of collecting their own at this stage.

Allow at least a further month before final release, or winter over if late in the year, and effect the release as for adult casualties. (see special note in Appendix A).

Grey
squirrel

Red
squirrel

13

Stoats, Weasels and similar

Four species are featured in this group – the stoat, the weasel, the polecat and the pine marten. All belong to the same family and all resemble (with variations in size and colour) the domestic ferret to which they are all closely related. The elongated body is the principal feature, together with rather short legs (somewhat longer in the case of the pine marten). The weasel is the smallest in length at about 10in. (25cm) including tail, then the stoat, polecat and the pine marten at about 27in. (67.5cm). In colouring the stoat and the weasel are very similar with brown on top and white beneath and, in some regions, both can change their coats to completely white in winter with the stoat retaining a black tail tip – the distinguishing feature between the two species. For many years, the poor old stoat has been called upon to sacrifice its winter coat for trimming the robes of lords and dignitaries, where it is called ermine. It is, after all, much more dignified to have robes trimmed with ermine than with stoat!

The polecat is dark brown to black with a sort of creamy-yellow under fur showing through and white around the face. It's very seldom found now in this country, although still quite common in the rest of Europe, and must be considered as rare. The pine marten is the largest of the four species under discussion, and is even rarer in this country than the polecat. It has longer legs than the others, and is darkish brown in colouring with a creamy-yellow bib.

As well as being trapped for fur, the group suffer great persecution from gamekeepers and poultry farmers, as they will take the charges of both of these. They can only be beneficial to the rest of the farming community and foresters, as they kill rabbits and a great many rodents. The pine marten also disposes of squirrels which pleases the foresters.

It is always difficult to plead the case for continuing existence of an animal which people seldom (if ever) see. 'If we never see it,' they might say, 'what difference does it make if it isn't there at all?' From a purely aesthetic point of view, there is no answer to this. You can't see any less of an animal which becomes extinct if you never saw it when it existed! But, ecologically, there is always a difference. When a species is wiped out, it could lead to the decimation or proliferation of one or more other species which in turn can have quite cataclysmic effects. Pine martens used to be quite common, but their extinction in most parts of the country has undoubtedly led to the great success of the grey squirrel, which is currently defying all attempts at artificial control.

Possible Handling Hazards

All of this group have a very respectable bite and are inclined to hang on when they have bitten. As with most wild animals, they will prefer to run from a human but this group are prepared to put up a fight if necessary and are very quick, lithe and agile. The long body is very supple and can be bent head to tail so that the teeth can catch you at most points where you might make a grab.

Approach and Capture

The chances of encountering an incapacitated member of this group are fairly remote but if it should happen, a pair of fairly stout gloves would be distinctly advantageous. Take a quick, firm hold just behind the head with the hand encircling the neck and forequarters. Lifting the animal from the ground in this manner, there is no way it can bite the handler, and providing the neck is not squeezed, there is no danger to the animal itself. In the case of a weasel or possibly even a stoat, a bird-catching net (Fig. 1) might be employed to save having to handle the animal at all or, failing anything else, the 'throw a coat over it' routine could be employed.

Transportation

We have never come across or had brought to us an injured member of this group, nor have we ever seen a dead one at the roadside. As a result, the information in this and subsequent parts of the chapter is, to some extent, speculative and is based on experience with tame and captive animals.

Members of the group are not inclined to use their teeth as an aid to escape from a container although they may, if fit enough to do so, scratch with their front feet in the manner of a dog digging. This is rather ineffectual, however, and a sack should be sufficient to contain the animal for a short journey. For a long distance, a wooden box or a wicker cat basket should fill the bill, so long as you remember that these animals can get through a hole much smaller than might be imagined. Virtually anywhere the head will fit through, the body will too.

Initial Care

Your patient is unlikely to chew the fixtures and fittings and can therefore be kept in any kind of room or shed but in selecting where it should be kept, the expression 'stink like a polecat' is relevant. All of the group possess scent glands from which they can emit odour and in the case of the polecat, it is pungent, to say the least. The stoat's scent too could be described as moderately horrible in a confined space!

Ensure there are no holes through which escape can be effected and this includes windows. The group are all good climbers so ensure there is nothing up which they can climb to reach an open window. Apart from indulging in a bit of digging action – which is more likely to be in the water bowl than at a possible point of egress – your patient will probably not be too perturbed by a captive state and should eat readily and heartily.

Food

The pine marten is known to eat a few berries occasionally, but apart from this the whole group is carnivorous. Dead day-old chicks, if you can get hold of any (see Chapter 5), will be devoured with alacrity and, if a regular supply can be obtained, could form the principal item of diet. Virtually anything 'fish, flesh or fowl' is likely to meet with an enthusiastic response and this does literally include fish which will tickle the palate of most. Tinned dog meat can be used whenever there is nothing else suitable, and a bowl of milk will be lapped up with delight. An occasional raw egg will also go down very well. There is unlikely to be any fastidious sniffing and picking. This is a group which tucks into its food with evident lip-smacking enjoyment, leaving nothing on the plate, and any failure to do so is likely to indicate serious internal problems.

Force-feeding

Not a very practical proposition.

Symptoms, Diagnosis and Treatment

Stoats and weasels are rarely seen and tend to hide themselves away when sick and injured. They may, however, be found in snares and traps but usually dead. They are semi-nocturnal, get caught at night and will struggle continuously – to the death – to get free. If found alive the injuries are frequently too severe to heal, and the animal should be taken to a veterinary surgeon to be put to sleep humanely.

General Care

An enclosure such as an aviary, so long as it is covered with very small mesh netting, would be suitable to house one of this group out of doors – but obviously not with birds in residence at the same time. Provide some sort of house where the animal can retire during its sleeping periods and can also shelter from bad weather. A wooden box, raised slightly off the ground and covered over with a sheet of plastic or roofing felt would suffice. Bear in mind that these animals are good climbers so the enclosure must also have a top covering. Even the overhang recommended for a fox enclosure (see Chapter 14) may not deter one of these agile characters.

Release

A weasel can be released virtually anywhere in the country (except Ireland where it is not found) and will readily find a niche. The stoat too has a general distribution which includes Ireland, whereas the other members of the group must now be considered rare and very localized. The polecat has its main remaining stronghold in Wales, and the pine marten is restricted to parts of the Lake District, parts of the north of England, Wales, Scotland and Ireland. It would, of course, be most unfair to release any animal where others of its species are not found, consequently the release of a polecat or pine marten should only be carried out in consultation with someone who can tell you just where the particular species is to be found if it can't be released in the area it came from.

Although all of the group come out during the day from time to time, they should be considered as nocturnal animals and released at dusk.

Orphans

It is most unlikely you will meet a suckling infant of one of this group, although an occasional youngster just past the weaning stage is found or carried in by a cat.

Try the youngster first to see if it can lap, on a half and half mixture of milk and water. If it can, provide a constant supply in a low dish, also some sloppy meat such as tinned dog meat mixed with a little diluted milk. A pinch of glucose added to the milk will be beneficial.

If the youngster cannot yet lap, feed as for baby rabbits (Chapter 11), but always put down a small quantity of solid food, changing it for fresh each day, as you will not be sure when your infant will be ready to take it. A shallow dish of milk should also be provided and bottle feeding should continue for at least a week *after* the infant has started to lap, albeit in reduced quantities, as it will not, at first, be getting enough to sustain it.

The nursery too should be as Chapter 11, see pages 103-4.

When the infant is fully furred and active and has been eating and drinking for at least two weeks, it can be transferred outside but do provide warm bedding in the sleeping box – hay, for instance. Retain in the enclosure until the autumn or possibly even over to the following spring to give the animal a good start, although the animal may well be too dependant by that time for a release to a completely wild existence. The odd one or two we have reared have been past the bottle stage when they came in. They were not handled unduly, and retained an air of independence. Incidentally, these have only been weasels.

In general, if the animal can be released directly from the enclosure in which it has been living, we would recommend giving it a try, while continuing to provide food in the enclosure to which it has free access.

It is by no means an unusual occurrence to come across a ferret, the domesticated member of this group, which has gone astray during the rabbiting operations for which ferrets are widely used. Strangely enough, although the ferret is an efficient killer like the rest of the group, it does not usually fare well when out on its own. We have them brought to us frequently and they are almost invariably in very poor bodily condition on arrival.

There is less likelihood of being bitten by a ferret than by another member of the group since they are usually accustomed to being handled. But, nevertheless, the same precautions should be taken when handling. House and feed your ferret patient as already described.

There is yet another relative which may be found, namely, the American mink, many of which have escaped from mink farms. The mink is similar to the ferret but is usually a uniform very dark brown in colour as opposed to the ferret's creamy or polecat colouring. The mink is deadly to virtually every indigenous species of up to its own size and even larger. It should on no account be released to the wild in this country.

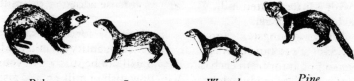

Polecat   Stoat   Weasel   Pine marten

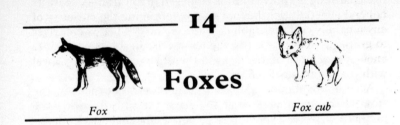

14

Foxes

Fox   *Fox cub*

We hear some very strange identifications from time to time. For instance 'a duck with a long neck and long legs' turns out to be a bittern, or a red deer hind is described as 'a thin brown donkey'. In the case of the fox there should be no such confusion. Although many people have never seen a fox 'in the flesh', it is extremely unlikely that anyone would fail to recognize the adult animal.

Small cubs, however, bear little resemblance to their parents. They have a grey coat instead of the adult red, rather flat faces, and stringy little tails which give no hint of the magnificent brushes they will become. On one occasion we almost came to blows with a man who brought in a small dead animal for us to identify. He had already informed press and television – presumably with visions of triumphant appearances as the finder of some hitherto unknown species – and was most upset when we told him that his 'find' was a fox cub. He snatched back the little body declaring that we didn't know what we were talking about and stormed from the premises. We subsequently learned that he had called on the local museum curator, the County Naturalists' Trust and Bristol Zoo in an endeavour to obtain a more exotic identification.

The saying 'give a dog a bad name' could have been devised especially for the fox, who is blamed for just about everything short of bank robbery, even though much of the evidence doesn't stand up to close scrutiny. It is often claimed, for instance, that foxes kill domestic cats. We have never encountered a single authenticated case of this having happened. On the contrary, what we *have* seen is a film (taken by Eric Ashby in the New Forest) of a fox and a cat passing one another, albeit warily, along a path. The fox isn't noted for its bravery and it is extremely unlikely it would attack a cat, which would make a formidable adversary. There are many easier pickings, and if the fox is not brave, it is undoubtedly resourceful and adaptable.

Another piece of 'foxlore' of doubtful authenticity is that of a fox 'charming' its prey. The fox is alleged to roll around, chase its tail and generally act the fool thereby engaging the curiosity of any mentally deficient rabbits in the vicinity. The fox contrives to gradually move closer to the mesmerised rabbits until close enough to pounce on the nearest, thereby securing a tasty meal with the minimum of effort.

Accusations abound of attacks on lambs and, occasionally, the stomach contents of a dead fox have certainly revealed the presence of wool. Eye-witness accounts of actual attacks, however, are seemingly non-existent. So, while not entirely ruling out the possibility of such an attack on rare occasions, we consider it much more likely that the lambs are usually dead or dying and have been abandoned by the ewe before the fox appears on the scene.

It cannot be denied that a fox will wreak havoc in a chicken house. Many would (and do) say this is pure blood lust, though a more plausible explanation would surely be instinctive opportunism, directing the animal to provide for more than its immediate needs when the chance is offered. The fox regularly hides voles, for instance, that it doesn't immediately need to eat, to dig up later when times are lean. We ourselves go off into town and buy up enough food to last a week or more and consider this to be perfectly rational behaviour. What's so different about the fox attempting to do the same?

Possible Handling Hazards

Although there is nothing wrong with its dental equipment, a fox is unlikely to offer the direct jaw-clamping bite a dog might inflict. There will be no attempt to bite at all until a hand is almost touching and even then it will only be a glancing snap, often accompanied by a terrified yelp as it attempts to escape.

Approach, Capture and Transportation

It is reasonable to assume that there is something wrong with any fox which fails to move off quickly. As with most wildlife casualties, the fox will try to reach hiding, even if only partially mobile, and this can help to gather up a casualty. A tea chest or similar sized wooden box will make a suitable travelling container. If the animal can move at all and the box is placed in his line of retreat with the opening towards him and a sack or cloth over most of the opening, it may well appear a welcome haven. He can be encouraged to go in the right direction with the aid of one or two large pieces of flat board in the manner of herding pigs, preventing it escaping to the side.

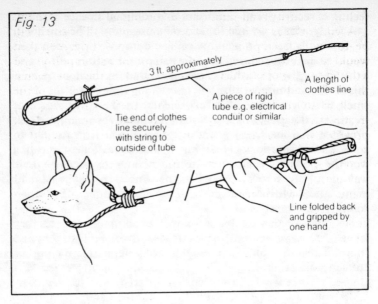

Fig. 13

3 ft. approximately

A piece of rigid tube e.g. electrical conduit or similar

A length of clothes line

Tie end of clothes line securely with string to outside of tube

Line folded back and gripped by one hand

It may prove necessary to lift the animal and then the use of a dog grasper (Fig. 13) is recommended since this removes all possibility of a bite. If such an implement, or the materials to make one, are not available, one hand (preferably gloved) should be moved slowly, but in full view, towards the animal's nose. When it makes a snap, this hand is withdrawn and the other hand takes a very firm grasp of the scruff. Normally, once a fox feels itself firmly held in this manner it will make no further attempt to struggle. Maintaining the grasp on the scruff, the free hand can be employed to lift the casualty into the container. This operation is not as difficult as it sounds. The fox is not a very strong animal and this, coupled with its tendency to lie dormant when held, means that a grip on its scruff is easier to maintain than on a terrier dog. The weaker hand – the left hand of a right-handed person – should be the 'bait', and a better grip can be achieved if the gripping hand is bare.

Initial Care

Wherever the fox is to be accommodated, it is a sound idea to allow it to keep the travelling container as a substitute 'earth'. The less chopping and changing the better, and the container will already feel comforting and familiar by the time the destination is reached, no matter how short the journey. A feeling of security is all-important to the animal's peace of mind.

A wild fox does *not* make the ideal house-guest. The smell will be, to say the least, pungent. A garage, outhouse or garden shed would be best to accommodate the patient for a short period and a thick covering of sawdust is recommended for the floor (even if this is changed regularly, it will take a long time to get rid of the smell when your guest has departed!). In the early stages of treatment, the garage or shed will be adequate for an injured fox, provided that everyone in the neighbourhood isn't invited to come and have a look. However, in the convalescent stages a wooden shed may not do since some foxes will try to chew their way out. This is by no means standard practice. We have had many foxes which have made no such attempt, even when confined for quite lengthy periods. But there is no way of knowing in advance whether or not your particular fox will be a 'chewer' so keep a careful watch. A few slivers of wood gnawed from a doorpost is sufficient warning that a change to chew-proof accommodation is needed.

Food

Catering is quite easy, for the average fox will take readily to tinned dog or cat food and, indeed, will eat most kitchen scraps. As a regular diet, while in captivity, tinned dog meat mixed with dog biscuit will be perfectly satisfactory, and the quantity should be the same as that recommended on the tin for a dog of comparable size to the fox. One feed per day is sufficient for an adult and, if the food fails to disappear, the fox's mouth and jaw should be examined for injury as most foxes could be described as 'good trenchermen' even in the most adverse circumstances.

A bowl of clean water should be available at all times and inspected frequently, for many foxes, for reasons best known to themselves, urinate in their water bowls. This can be somewhat trying when you've just washed the bowl and provided nice clean water, particularly if you've had to carry it some distance. They don't all do it so you might be lucky enough to have one with more decorum.

If there should be any temporary feeding problems, but the animal can still lap, milk and any kind of baby cereal will be most acceptable or even a good thick meat soup.

Force-feeding foxes is inadvisable.

Symptoms, Diagnosis and Treatment

A fox that is sick or injured will invariably try to return to its earth or go into hiding to 'lick its wounds'. It is likely, therefore, that those foxes which are come across are the worst cases, needing much treatment, care and attention. If they are too badly injured or diseased, it may be kinder to put them to sleep to cut short their suffering.

The commonest causes of disability are road accidents, capture in snares or traps, poisoning and disease.

Injuries. Road accidents are not uncommon, for though the fox is intelligent and fast on his feet, and he has discovered that the car will not usually chase him through hedges and across fields – or if it does it is not as persistent in pursuit as the horse and hound – he often misjudges the speed. The majority of accident injuries are to the rear end of the animals – cuts and bruises, and fractures of limbs, pelvis and spine. Of course some are struck on the body, and head and neck region. In addition to bruising and laceration, many suffer internal injuries, perhaps haemorrhage and shock. From a recent study of over three hundred foxes killed in London in various ways, ninety-one had healed fractures. Twenty-four had broken ribs, forty-two had fractures of the spine and tail, sixteen involved the pelvis, twenty-nine involved the hind limb, and twenty-three the fore limb. Altogether 41 per cent involved the forequarters and 59 per cent the hindquarters.

Broken legs can be diagnosed by their awkward appearance. The limb bends where there is no joint and often a grating noise can be heard when it is moved. There is often damage to the skin which may be broken and bleeding. If major limb bones are fractured the animal is unable to use the limb and will drag it. In the fore limb this can be confused with paralysis caused by damage to the radial nerve. When minor limb bones are affected the animal can move the limb but is obviously in pain and will not usually walk on it. It limps visibly by throwing its head up when the affected limb touches the ground, and comes down heavily on the normal limb.

Fractures of the pelvis cause various symptoms depending on the site of the break. In some cases, apart from pain little can be observed. In other cases the animal may have difficulty in walking and may sway awkwardly from side to side.

Fractures of the spine usually cause a great deal of pain and if the spinal cord (the nerve trunk running down the spine) is nipped or damaged there could be loss of feeling below or behind the injury.

Internal injuries, such as damage to the liver, are difficult to diagnose. The mucous membranes of the eye and mouth become pale or blueish if there is internal bleeding. But this is also a symptom of shock.

Capture in snares and traps has become more frequent because fox skins can be sold. Snares often catch the fox around the neck, or neck and one fore leg, causing strangulation and severe damage to skin and tissues. The poor animal, finding itself caught, pulls and tugs to escape. The snare tightens and the animal may lose consciousness and collapse. The snare may then go slack and the creature regains consciousness to begin its struggles again. If the fox is caught by its leg it usually struggles till the wire cuts deeply into or through the limb.

Traps cause as much damage, not only inflicting severe lacerations, but the trapped animal sometimes chews off its foot in its efforts to escape. Often the skin is stripped off and the bones are exposed.

Diseases and Poisoning. The symptoms of poisoning depend on the type of poison used. Strychnine causes periodic simultaneous contractions of all the muscles, producing cramp-like pain. The exterior muscles are more powerful so the animal's limbs are extended, the back bent concavely with the head thrown back, and the facial muscles pulled tight. After a few seconds the muscles relax. Any small stimulus will cause contraction again. Gradually the contraction periods get longer and the interval of relaxation less until the animal dies of asphyxia. *The use of strychnine for all mammals except moles is illegal.*

The other common type of poisoning is by pesticides such as Malathion or Parathion, which belong to a group called organo-phosphorus compounds. These substances act on insects and animals by interfering with the action of an enzyme in the nervous system, which causes a state of chaos. The symptoms are depression, muscular weakness, diarrhoea and eventually prost-ration. Symptoms appear within twenty-four hours of exposure, and last several days. Smaller doses cause chronic poisoning, muscular twitching, loss of weight, and diarrhoea that may persist for weeks.

Warfarin poisoning sometimes occurs because foxes occasion-ally eat meal in which the poison is laid, usually for rats. It interferes with the clotting mechanism of the blood and produces symptoms of weakness, bloody diarrhoea, and haemorrhage throughout the body muscles, particularly over bony promin-ences, and in the joints, which causes lameness.

Foxes are susceptible to canine diseases and a sick, thin, depressed-looking fox may be suffering from one of these. However, if the animal can be approached there is probably little hope that treatment will produce a cure.

In Europe foxes are responsible for the spread of rabies – which can infect any mammal. But due to our strict quarantine laws there is no rabies in Britain at the moment and therefore *no* danger that the fox may spread it.

The most common disease in foxes is mange – a skin infection caused by a minute spider-like creature called sarcoptes. It is transmitted by contact and gradually spreads over the animal's body causing loss of hair and a thickening of the skin.

Treatment of the more serious accidents, trap and snare injuries, and poisoning and diseases should be left to a veterinary surgeon. First aid can be given, however – wounds bandaged, haemorrhage stopped by placing a pad of gauze on the bleeding point and binding it tight enough to occlude the vessel, shock treated by protecting the animal from cold and keeping it quiet. Though veterinary treatment is usually necessary it is only part of the story. Good nursing and after-care are essential to success. It is interesting that the fox is much less persistent than the domestic dog in chewing and worrying at the bandage or plaster. Very often the fox will completely ignore it.

The treatment the veterinary surgeon will use for fractures varies with the bone that is broken and the type of fracture. In some cases it may be sufficient to bandage the area, others may require a plaster cast, while some can be 'pinned' with metal rods or plates. The vet will probably suture nearly all wounds and may give the animal a shot of long-acting antibiotic. If a paw is badly injured part of it may be amputated. But because the fox will eventually be released, nothing is usually done that will seriously reduce his future ability to capture his food.

Strychnine poisoning can often be successfully treated by a vet for the poison does not persist indefinitely in the animal's body. The usual treatment is to keep the animal relaxed under anaesthesia (usually barbiturate) until the poison has been dealt with by the animal's metabolic processes.

Pesticide persists for a long time and interferes with the animal's automatic function and the prognosis is less hopeful.

Mange can be treated with one of the special insecticide dressings provided the disease does not cover too much of the animal's body, for the dressing is poisonous. It must be applied at regular intervals, over five to seven days, as one treatment is not enough.

General Care

If the fox needs to be kept for a prolonged period an outdoor pen is desirable and this should be constructed of material rather stronger than ordinary wire netting – Twilweld of at least 16 gauge, or chain link with a mesh size about 2 × 2in. (50 × 50mm), is most satisfactory. But it must be remembered that a fox can (and will) both dig and climb. It will scale a wire mesh fence with consummate ease but will be completely baffled by an overhang of about 18in. (45cm) (Fig. 14). To counter any digging, similar wire mesh must be placed on the ground covering about 40in. (1 metre) all round the inside of the perimeter and firmly fixed to the bottom of the fence. It is *not* necessary to cover the whole ground area of the pen since the fox will invariably try to dig at the base of the fence. We have not yet encountered one resourceful enough to work out that in order to get under the fence, digging operations must commence a metre in from the base.

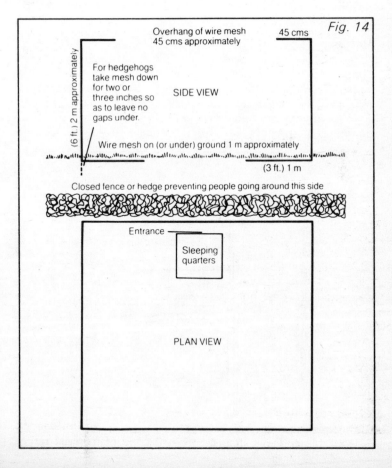

Fig. 14

A small house of some kind must be provided as an earth, just as in the indoor accommodation. The animal will not be unduly perturbed at the approach of people so long as it can rapidly get completely out of sight. For this reason, the entrance to the house must be set in such a way that anyone approaching cannot see into it and cannot reach that side of the pen (Fig. 15). If the original travelling box is still serviceable, it can be made reasonably weatherproof with the addition of a sheet of plastic over the top and sides, and it should be used in preference to a new residence. To paraphrase an old saying, 'familiarity breeds content'.

There is no easy way to keep an outside pen clean and odour free unless it is concrete based and can be swilled regularly. A foul-smelling pen may quickly undermine the sympathy and tolerance of neighbours so place the pen as far away as possible from their houses.

Release

Release of an adult casualty must be at the earliest possible moment consistent with a reasonable chance of survival. There is an understandable tendency among wildlife first-aiders to hold onto patients longer than necessary, doubting their ability to cope again with the rough and tumble of life in the wild. If in doubt, it is probably time for the animal to go and take its

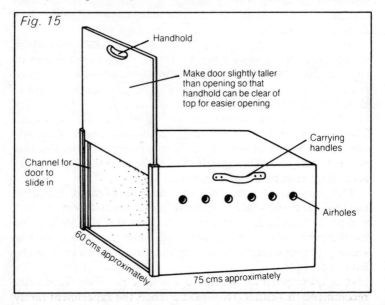

Fig. 15

Handhold

Make door slightly taller than opening so that handhold can be clear of top for easier opening

Carrying handles

Channel for door to slide in

Airholes

60 cms approximately

75 cms approximately

chances. There is little likelihood of a fox caught as an adult becoming imprinted (see *Orphans*), but prolonged captivity may well dull the sharp edge of awareness necessary to survive in the wild.

If release can be effected on the animal's home ground, this in itself will contribute to its chances of survival but the fox is very adaptable and will quickly find a niche in almost any situation.

Orphans

If a normally wild animal is not afraid of people, someone will undoubtedly kill it unless it is living in a sheltered environment, a sad reflection on the human race. Fox cubs are quite easy to rear, but imprinting (losing the fear of and becoming dependent on humans) is a major problem, particularly when there is only one cub to be reared.

Finding a solitary infant of a species which normally produces more than one (a fox litter averages four) gives grounds for suspicion that there may be something wrong which has caused the parent to reject and abandon this particular offspring, although there may be nothing readily apparent. We had a fox cub brought to us on one occasion with its eyes only just opening which meant that it was no more than two weeks old (the eyes open for the first time at about ten days). We could find nothing wrong and set about rearing the cub. About three weeks later, we realized it was mentally deficient. It would seem the vixen had detected something amiss much earlier than we did.

Before undertaking the rearing of fox cubs, the implications should be fully appreciated, not least of which is the length of time they will have to be kept. In the wild, assuming they have not been dug out earlier, fox cubs will emerge from their earth at about the beginning of May, when they are around four weeks old. It is at this time of year that most stray cubs are picked up. They would part from the vixen, in the normal course of events, during late August or early September, and we consider that this is when those reared in captivity should be released – so a stay of some four months is the minimum.

The prospect of a fox cub imprinted on humans returning successfully to the wild is very remote. Having no fear of humans will prove a fatal affliction even if the animal is able to fend for itself. For this reason, we do not recommend that anyone should attempt to rear a single fox cub unless it is intended to keep the animal as a pet.

It is quite possible to keep a fox as a pet, but we do not recommend this either. In our experience, the experiment rarely succeeds. A fox does not take at all kindly to being moved from one home to another (during holidays, etc.) and more often than not the animal eventually has to be destroyed. Our advice, if you find yourself in possession of a single cub, is to try and find someone else in similar circumstances, possibly via the local RSPCA Inspector, County Naturalists' Trust or even the local news media, and to raise the cubs together. They needn't be from the same family; we regularly rear groups of up to a dozen all from different families and from different parts of the country. Ideally, more than one person should be involved in the rearing as will be explained.

If the cubs are too young to feed themselves – if they have been dug out, we would recommend feeding on Sherley's Lactol, obtainable from most pet shops, following the instructions for quantities and frequency of feeding for puppies which are on the side of every tin. A plastic syringe without the needle is useful for administering it. Always leave a dish of Lactol on the floor as well since the cubs will start helping themselves much sooner than you would think from their size. As soon as they are able to lap, provide a dish of solid food also. Tinned dog meat mixed with puppy meal biscuit will serve quite satisfactorily.

It must be remembered that if the cubs are from different litters, they will not necessarily be of the same age, so care must be taken that they can *all* feed themselves before the bottle/syringe feeding is finished.

If possible, when weaning is completed, the person who has been doing the bottle feeding of the cubs, and therefore the handling, should drop out of the scene and never go near them again. This is because there will have been a measure of imprinting caused by the handling and bottle feeding but, at this stage, hopefully only on that one person. The person taking over after weaning must *never* handle the cubs and, indeed, must frighten them off should they venture near.

Cubs should be provided with a dark box for an 'earth' to which they can run and hide. The box need not be very large as they seem to prefer it snug so that they can pack in like sardines. We have found a box $30 \times 24 \times 24$in. ($75 \times 60 \times 60$cm) approximately is sufficient for up to five cubs, even when they are quite well grown. The box should be portable with some means of closing the entrance when the cubs are inside with adequate ventilation when closed. The reason for this will become apparent later.

After weaning, one good meal a day is all that is necessary, and the more squabbling and fighting over it the better. We use mainly dead day-old chicks from a local hatchery, and even dead-in-shell chicks which we feed complete with shell. The idea, held by some, that this will give the cubs a taste for poultry is quite erroneous. Foxes have a taste for virtually anything edible, and a steady diet of chicks does not preclude their falling upon anything else which might come within reach. Nor will it give them a preference for chicks over other food, as they will eat anything that involves them in the minimum of effort.

Fresh water should always be available, although foxes do not appear to drink a great deal. The earlier remarks about the unsavoury habits of some adult foxes with their water bowls also applies to cubs, with the added refinement that some cubs are apt to defaecate in them too, just for good measure!

By the time of release, indeed from the time of the second person taking over, the cubs should be ready and willing to bite the hand that feeds them and should flee to the safety of their 'earth' at the approach of any human. They should also have the strongest possible objection to being handled or molested in any way.

There are two ways in which release can be effected, neither of which involves any handling. The first is simply to open the door of the pen, allowing the cubs to make their own way into the world beyond. Continue putting food into the pen so that they can return for a meal should they wish to do so. Although this is undoubtedly the best way to release them, in most cases it simply isn't practicable for one reason or another.

The second way is to shut the cubs in their box when they run in to hide (hence the door) and transport them to the point of release. This should be as far away as possible from human habitation and preferably in a piece of rough woodland. The permission of the landowner must be given first, of course. The box should if possible be left at the release point and the release effected by just opening the door. The box will afford the cubs an orientation point and if food can be left in the vicinity for several days, so much the better. There will be no way of knowing whether or not it is the cubs who are eating the food, unless there is someone who can spare the time to keep watch, but it *may* just help them to get started on their independent lives.

The cubs will not remain where they are released and will quickly have to face all of the hazards which are the price of a free-living existence. At least you'll know you've done the best you can, the rest is up to them. We have reared and released many cubs in the manner described and, from observations made, believe it to be a successful formula.

15

Otters

Books such as *Tarka the Otter* and *Ring of Bright Water* have done much to carve out a place in the affections of most people for this lively, playful, and altogether delightful little animal, in spite of the fact that few people have ever seen one at all, and even less have actually seen one in its wild state. It seems now quite incredible that the otter, which has for some years been hovering on the brink of extinction in this country, was being hunted with packs of hounds as recently as December 1977. The human race surely has a lot to answer for.

In appearance, the otter is superficially similar to a stoat or a weasel and it does, in fact, belong to the same family. It is, however, a much larger animal reaching up to 4 feet (1.2m) or so in length including the tail which makes up roughly a third of the length. The tail is cylindrical in shape and very thick and powerful, being the animal's main propulsion unit when swimming. Further aid in this respect is provided by webbed feet which allow the otter great manoeuvrability under water, making it a comfortable match for most fish.

The otter is agile both in and out of the water and can move rapidly in both elements – attributes not enjoyed by many other indigenous creatures (which are apt to be rather clumsy in one or the other). But it is in the water that the otter really seems at home and is at its most graceful, diving and twisting with a flick of the tail as it pursues a fish – or simply with pure *joie de vivre*.

Apart from being hunted, a number of things have contributed to the otter's precipitous decline. Being a shy, elusive and sensitive creature, it hasn't taken kindly to the recent great increase in the use of waterways for many and diverse leisure pursuits. Pesticides draining from fields into streams, and a thousand and one other kinds of pollution flowing indiscriminately into rivers, do not help in providing a viable environment. Nor does the draining of marshlands – now being done on a grand scale – which is a disaster for many other wild creatures besides the otter.

In the past twenty or so years, vast strides have been made in the cleaning-up of waterways and the monitoring of what goes into them. Unfortunately this very clean-up which should, on the face of it, provide an altogether happier outlook for the otter, has instead generated a vast increase in human use of waterways. To use the old saying, the poor old otter seems to be 'on a hiding to nothing'.

Possible Handling Hazards

It would be more correct to head this section *probable* handling hazards. Any attempt to actually handle an adult otter in possession of all its faculties, even with the use of thick gloves, would be most foolhardy and would almost certainly result in one or more very severe bites, with the loss of one or more fingers a distinct risk (and the subsequent loss of a hand not beyond the bounds of possibility). The otter's body is very supple as well as being very strong, able to reach virtually any part of its anatomy with its formidable teeth, so there is no place it can be grabbed with impunity.

Approach and Capture

If the animal is mobile, the chances of approach are minimal. It is therefore only one with a moderate to severe injury which is likely to be encountered – although with only an estimated 200 in the whole of England and Wales (rather more in Scotland and Ireland), the chances of such an encounter are very remote. For this same reason, if one *should* be found, every effort should be made to save it and return it to the wild where every individual animal is of the utmost importance if the species is not to become totally extinct in this country.

An otter can be lifted with a dog catcher but not around the neck. The noose must go over both neck and forequarters (front legs) otherwise it is most likely to just slip off when an attempt is made to lift. When the animal is in the travelling container, the noose can easily be released by allowing the line to slide right through the handle (from the handle end). It can be re-threaded later.

An alternate method is to tangle the animal up in a piece of heavy netting of any sort which might come to hand, taking care to keep the hands well clear. This will allow for a veterinary surgeon to administer an anaesthetic through the netting without much danger of being bitten and the otter can then be untangled for an inspection either prior to, or after, the journey.

If no dog grasper or netting are available, a table cloth or sheet might be eased under the animal with two people holding the edge taut and using a sort of sawing action. Once the patient is on the cloth, it can then be lifted by the corners and both the cloth and the patient deposited in the travelling container.

Transportation

A wood or metal container is preferable but failing that a sack will probably suffice for the journey. Otters are not inclined to make much of a fuss when in a container and an injured one will welcome the seclusion.

Initial Care

An otter will be unlikely to chew at the woodwork or demolish the fixtures and fittings although it may attack any exposed electric wires (which should be well out of reach). If a suitable bolt-hole is provided such as a tea chest placed on its side with the open end facing a wall and about 9in. (22cm) away from it, and the open end partly covered with a sack or cloth, the otter will doubtless be grateful for this and will be happy to keep out of sight. With these provisos, any room can be used as a temporary residence (although obviously a bit of a mess will be made on the floor so don't endanger your best Persian carpet!).

Food

The otter is quite a good trencherman consuming about 20lb (9–10kg) of food per week in the wild. Items on the menu include fish – principally chub and roach, as well as sticklebacks and other small ones – frogs, newts, the odd duckling, rabbits and small rodents. When 'summering' at the seaside, crabs and sundry other creatures found in the shallows are high on the list of favourite delicacies, but taking precedence over all others, are eels. The average otter will sell its soul for an eel so in captivity, chopped or whole eels are an obvious appetite tempter. Other items which can be offered are minced raw beef, whiting, and dead day-old chicks. Water should, of course, also be provided.

Symptoms, Diagnosis and Treatment

Though extremely playful, otters do occasionally bite each other and probably because the animal is continually in water, wounds tend to turn septic. In captivity, wounds should be kept clean and antibiotics administered daily.

Not infrequently, an abcess may develop inside the mouth. If it is very large the animal should be anaesthetized, the abcess opened and drained, and a course of antibiotics given until it has healed. Smaller abcesses may be treated with antibiotics alone.

A mouth abcess is dangerous because, should it burst in the mouth, there is a danger of the otter inhaling the pus and causing pneumonia. This disease is not uncommon in otters, probably because it is constantly in water. Anything that damages the coat and allows water to penetrate may lead to pneumonia. The animal stops eating, its coat becomes dishevelled and unkempt, and the eyes become dull and watery. Later there may be a discharge from the nose.

These symptoms also occur, however, with leptospirosis, a disease of the kidneys and liver.

General Care

When convalescent, an otter should really have access to a pool as well as a large outdoor paddock and it is most unlikely, short of a considerable financial outlay, that the average person could provide suitable temporary accommodation at this stage in the proceedings. Indeed, owing to the scarcity of the species and the dire need to save every one possible, we would recommend that an otter be passed on, as soon as possible, to somewhere fully equipped and experienced to offer it the optimum possible chance of survival. The Otter Trust in Suffolk (see Appendix D) is such a place. Holding onto *any* animal which might have better prospects elsewhere can only be construed as self-indulgence. Holding onto one so rare in such circumstances is not what this book is about.

Release

Otters range over quite long distances so, if one is picked up injured, it is extremely difficult to judge just where it was coming from or going to. If it is found during a hot summer when streams are getting a bit low, it was probably on its way to the seaside. As with other species which are thin on the ground, as much advice as possible should be taken before effecting a release.

Orphans

Otter cubs seem to be born at any time during the year so there is no set time when orphans may be encountered. Obviously, with so few adults around, the chances of coming across a youngster are remote, but it is not unknown. The usual cause in such a case is the parent being hit by a car and killed, leaving the youngster or youngsters wandering vaguely about not knowing what to do without mum to show them. Any picked up at this stage will be in the region of ten weeks old and quite able to survive happily on a solid diet with no necessity to bottle feed although a drop of Lactol (or similar) in a dish may well meet with approval.

The chances of youngsters coming to hand which need bottle feeding are even more remote and would depend on some calamitous circumstance affecting the actual nursery, known as a hover or holt. Should this occur, very young infants are unlikely to survive long enough on their own to come to the notice of a possible benefactor.

For their first few weeks, the infants are possibly slightly less robust than badger cubs of the same age but they can be treated in the same way for initial care and feeding. Badgers too belong to the same family (*mustelidae*) although they don't look much like the other members.

Hand-reared otter cubs are apt to become very tame which does not bode well for their prospects in the wild so, as with adults, it is imperative that any youngsters found should be handed on as quickly as possible to experts. There they can be given every opportunity for a possible self-sufficient existence or, failing that, then at least a reasonable quality of life.

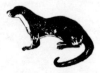

Otter

16

Marine Mammals

Around the coasts of the British Isles live quite a few marine mammals including two species of seal, and several species of dolphins and whales. The seals live and breed on various parts of the coast, on islands or in secluded coves, usually selecting sites not readily accessible to people. Whales and dolphins, although air-breathing mammals, never come ashore in normal circumstances.

The grey and the common are the two species of seal and, along with all other seals, are quite distinctive from any purely land-based mammal in general appearance. The main distinguishing feature is their lack of feet as such, which makes them very ungainly on land (although they can move faster than might be imagined). Few people would fail to recognize a seal, and the type of coastline where the sighting has taken place will give a further clue as to which of the two species it is. The common seal favours a low coastline with plenty of sandbanks, river estuaries and shallow areas in general, while the grey is much more at home on rocky coasts where there are cliffs, small inaccessible beaches and caves. The grey is also larger, up to about 10 feet (3m) in length, while the common reaches a maximum of only about 6 feet (1.8m).

Most people also have a fair idea as to what a dolphin and a whale look like. They've either seen them in captivity or on television, in one of the many good programmes of recent years which dealt with the plight of these highly intelligent creatures, abused and persecuted almost beyond belief. Apart from possible encounters at sea, these splendid animals become stranded from time to time. There are an average of about thirty such cases each year and the most common species involved are the common porpoise, the common dolphin, the bottle-nosed dolphin and the pilot whale, although other species such as the sperm whale can also be found. Not all of these animals are giants – the common porpoise, for instance, is only about 5 feet (1.5m) in length – but the pilot whale can reach a length of 28 feet (8.4m) – still quite modest by whale standards!

Possible Handling Hazards

There is little danger from a stranded whale or dolphin. They are completely helpless when well clear of the water and although all of those mentioned possess quite formidable teeth, only the most idiotic of persons is likely to suffer any damage from them. Seals on the other hand also have quite respectable dental equipment which they are not averse to using. Even the youngest of them will defend itself vigorously against any attempt at handling and very severe, possibly crippling, bites can result. There is a further danger from a seal bite in that it may result in a pathogenic infection requiring antibiotic treatment.

Approach and Capture

Approaching a stranded whale or dolphin is quite easy since the animal is unable to move and the question of 'capture' does not arise.

A seal should be approached from the rear and, if it is necessary to catch it, take hold only of the hind flippers. Nowhere else is really safe, even with a tiny pup.

Transportation

This is unlikely to arise in the case of whales and dolphins but, if it does, it is undoubtedly a matter for experts (see following section). It is a comparatively easy task to manoeuvre a small seal pup into a suitable container – which only need be a shallow box large enough to contain it comfortably, with no top being necessary since seals aren't very good at jumping! For an adult, a truck or van will be needed with a smooth ramp up which the animal can be hauled (see following section).

Initial Care

Before any question of transportation is attempted or even contemplated, it is essential to try and ascertain just why the animal is where it is. In the case of a seal, the animal may not require any help at all although if it is an adult or a well-grown pup and has come up on a beach not normally occupied by seals, the chances are there *is* something amiss pointing to possible sickness or injury. It may also have become badly contaminated with oil. Perfectly healthy pups which have recently reached self-sufficiency may occasionally come ashore on a strange beach, having exhausted themselves in the pursuit of a meal and, very infrequently, a pup may be born and reared on such a beach.

For an inexperienced person, it is very difficult to tell whether or not a particular seal needs help. Indeed, it isn't always easy for an experienced person, so we would strongly recommend the finder to seek a second opinion before taking any action. A call to the local RSPCA Inspector would be a sound idea, and if he doesn't attend to it himself, he will more than likely know the right person to call.

There is no certainty as to the reason or reasons why whales and dolphins become stranded. One possibility is that the animal may be seeking safety from drowning. Being air-breathing mammals, this can of course happen. Unlike land mammals, their breathing is not automatic but under conscious control, and if the animal should feel itself losing consciousness, it may seek shallow water in order to keep its blowhole above the surface. In some parts of the world, beached whales have been found to have a parasitic worm in the inner ear which may have caused loss of balance and probably was extremely painful. Indeed many infected animals have serious self-inflicted injuries of the skin above the ear area, apparently caused by rubbing against jagged rocks. Some other beached whales have poisonous amounts of mercury in their bodies, which may have caused mental derangement. Some, apparently fit and healthy, are thought to have been following a school of fish inshore and inadvertently become stranded when the tide receded. Mass strandings sometimes occur and a possible cause is that one animal becomes sick and the others rally round to go to its aid.

If a live stranded whale or dolphin should be found, help should be sought by informing the coastguard, the local police, or the local RSPCA Inspector. Remember, these animals are classified as 'royal fish' – the property of the crown. While awaiting assistance, a certain amount of first aid can be given the animal just by keeping the skin wet, particularly the flippers and tail fluke, but care should be taken not to get any water into the blowhole. It is easier to keep the animal wet by covering the body with cloths and towels and wetting these, and if the sun should be strong, a temporary shelter could be erected to give some shade. They are sensitive creatures and disturbance and noise should be minimized and onlookers kept well away.

Food

Seals eat only fish and may devour some thrown to them but hand-feeding or force-feeding can be a hazardous business with an adult animal and should most emphatically be left to someone with experience. No attempt should be made to feed stranded whales or dolphins.

Injury and Illness

It is a comparatively rare occurrence for an adult seal to be picked up sick or injured but such cases *do* occur. Because of the hazardous nature of dealing with such a patient and the expensive accommodation needed for convalescence, we strongly recommend that the help of some establishment specializing in marine mammals be enlisted and the same should be the case with stranded whales or dolphins.

General Care
See above.

Release
Again, this should be left to someone with experience. That person may well make the wrong decision in a given case – nobody is infallible, as anyone working in the wildlife field would readily admit – but at least the animal might have a chance of survival and, if not, is likely to meet its end less painfully at the hands of an expert than those of a novice.

Oil Pollution
It is not uncommon for a seal's coat to become contaminated with oil but this is by no means as serious a problem as it is for a bird. In general, nothing need be done and the oil will simply 'weather' off without causing the animal much problem. If the contamination is so extensive as to impair the animal's swimming ability (which in turn would deny it food), the oil can be removed in a similar manner to that described for oiled seabirds. Apart from the handling dangers, which cannot be over-emphasized, the actual cleaning is easier than for a bird and need not be quite so meticulous.

Orphans
There are a number of establishments around the coast dealing with orphaned seal pups of both species, which employ varying methods to deal with the problem of feeding. These range from tube feeding a mixture with a very high fat content to approximate the mother's milk, to bottle feeding with various mixtures such as Complan and emulsified fish, to feeding solid fish from the outset.

Although there is no very hard evidence of long-term survival after release (or at least none that has to date come to our notice), this is not to suggest that the pups do not survive. As pointed out in the oiled seabirds chapter, evidence of long-term survival of any sea creature is difficult to come by.

All of the methods mentioned above seem to enjoy a measure of success as well as a measure of failure and most people engaged in the work agree that a great deal more work needs to be done for any firm conclusions to be reached.

As with adults, there is little point in an individual attempting to set up facilities to attempt the rearing of a single pup. It is much better to send it where there are already suitable facilities and people with some prior knowledge willing to undertake the rearing. As mentioned earlier, the local RSPCA Inspector, particularly those at coastal stations, will almost certainly have knowledge of the nearest place which will help. And again, as suggested in the previous chapter, holding onto an animal which might have better prospects elsewhere is not only self-indulgent but not what caring for wildlife is all about.

*Common
seal*

17

Badgers

Here is a shy, harmless animal which has suffered quite vicious persecution at the hands of the human race for many years, with not the slightest justification. There certainly *appears* to be evidence of bovine tuberculosis being spread to cattle by badgers (see *Symptoms, Diagnosis and Treatment*), but this in no way excuses the disgusting maltreatment meted out by badger diggers and their dogs. These despicable individuals, often acting under a cloak of great respectability, make us ashamed to be members of the human race. No matter how it may be presented, there can be no possible mitigation of their actions.

A very large section of the public have never seen a badger but would instantly recognize one if they did. Many would, however, be very surprised at the size of it, as it measures up to 2ft 6in. (75cm) in length or even longer, and weighs up to $3\frac{1}{2}$ stone (22kg). The head is the most recognizable part, with its distinctive black and white stripes.

The main reason why it isn't seen more often is, of course, because it is a nocturnal animal, going about its business when most of us are in bed. It is by no means unusual for a badger sett (burrow) to be in close proximity to houses without the occupants being aware of it. It seems strange that this should be the case with such shy animals, but in most cases, the setts were there long before the houses since setts are used for many years, and badgers are rather hard to move once they are established.

Badgers could not be described as killers, except by those wanting to justify digging them out. They aren't fast moving – surely the essential feature of a predator – and are very much in favour of the quiet life, eating what comes easily to snout, rather than trying to catch things. In fact they are more likely to flee when faced with a squawking, flapping bird than try to tackle it. They will certainly eat any very young animals which do not run away, digging out young rabbits for instance, but it is fair to say that any animal that can run, or can kick up a lot of fuss, is unlikely to be eaten by a badger.

Gamekeepers and the shooting fraternity in general (many of

whom are fanatical to the point of neurosis in defence of the birds they will later slaughter unmercifully) often accuse badgers of decimating the breeding stock, but this is quite untrue. Badgers have been known to live very close to the breeding pens without bothering the birds at all.

Like that other slow moving nocturnal creature, the hedgehog, badgers suffer greatly on the roads. If it is possible, without causing a hazard to following traffic, the thing to do when meeting a badger on the road at night is to stop the vehicle and turn off the headlights for a few moments to give the animal a chance to reach the verge. It isn't just way out in the country that you might encounter a badger – we had one in recently which was run down on the main street of a small town.

In general, the badger could be described as the countryside's dustman in that it removes a good deal of refuse as it bumbles along. Any dead carcase it finds, be it bird, mammal, reptile or amphibian, will be eaten as will any odd scraps left by picnickers. Its staple food for most of the year is earthworms, of which it eats vast quantities, and surely nobody could object to that, except perhaps the worms themselves!

Possible Handling Hazards

The badger is a strong animal with powerful jaws that can inflict serious injuries on the unwary human. The bite is capable of amputating a finger, and should it decide to hang on, it also has a tenacious grip which is virtually impossible to loosen without breaking the animal's jaw. In spite of this formidable equipment, the badger is not pugnacious and will only bite when very much provoked – by handling for instance. Apart from the odd fracas with other badgers, its demeanour is amiable and non-belligerent and geared only to defence. But in defence of her cubs, a sow will fight bravely in the face of overwhelming odds and will not submit until killed.

The badger is also equipped with long powerful claws. These are not for offence or defence, only for digging, but if you should happen to be scratched accidentally, you will certainly know about it!

Approach and Capture

Badgers seem to have a positive genius for getting themselves into awkward situations. In a recent case, for instance, one had managed to fall into one of those huge tanks on a sewage farm. The tank was almost empty but had just sufficient unsavoury sludge in the bottom to surely class the subsequent rescue as 'beyond the call of duty'! On another occasion a cover had been left off and a badger had fallen down a 15-foot deep (4.5-metre) manhole. It hadn't hurt itself, but was pacing about at the bottom of the shaft, obviously most annoyed. As we peered dubiously down the hole, the chap who had called us asked, 'Do you mind if I watch how you do it?' Note the wording of this – not 'Do you think you'll be *able* to do it?' Our abilities had apparently been taken for granted as though we must surely be equipped for just such an eventuality, and would say, 'Ah yes – this calls for the Acme Badger Rescue Kit Mark 2, with 15-foot drain attachment'.

The moral of these stories is that one cannot hope to be equipped for every eventuality, and improvisation is called for in most circumstances for which no simple guidelines can be drawn.

An injured badger, when approached, will usually crouch down with its nose to the ground and will not attempt to bite until actually touched. A dog grasper (Fig. 1) is a very useful tool. The noose can usually be eased over the head without any great objection from the animal, and although the head and neck are somewhat tapered which doesn't help in maintaining a firm hold, it is usually sufficient to lift the animal into a container with the additional support of a handful of loose skin on the back near the rump. There is quite a generous amount of loose skin on a badger's back and lifting in this way causes no apparent discomfort. For the few seconds that all four feet are off the ground, the badger is completely disorientated and will not attempt to struggle.

Do not rely on even the thickest gloves when handling a badger. The thickness needed to preclude any possibility of injury would also prevent any movement of the hand (which would rather defeat the object).

If no dog grasper is available, endeavour to hold the animal's head on the ground with a thick stick until a good handful of loose skin on the back can be grasped. Then make the lift just by the skin, but the operation must be executed with the utmost confidence if it is to succeed with no discomfort to the animal and no damage to the handler. If you lack this confidence (as you well may if you haven't done it before), wait until some help is available.

Assuming some measure of mobility, the badger *may* be induced to enter a container of its own accord as suggested for the fox (Chapter 14), but this is somewhat less likely with a badger which is apt to keep shying away from the container, using up its strength and possibly exacerbating the injury.

Transportation

A metal container such as an old tin trunk is recommended although a wooden one would probably serve for the journey. Don't forget to make air holes. Any kind of strong cage could also be used but a closed container is better in that the patient will prefer not to see or be seen and will travel more restfully this way.

Initial Care

Unless completely incapacitated, a badger will not take kindly to being shut in anywhere and will employ both tooth and claw to the limit on any part of the structure that appears vulnerable and likely to afford a means of escape. In the average house there is really nowhere suitable to house even a semi-active badger except a garage with metal doors, and even here it may well try to dig up a concrete floor until its claws are torn and bleeding. However, if it is essential the animal be retained, then you can only use the best available, and hope it does not fret too much with the unaccustomed confinement. Leave the travelling container as a 'bolt-hole' (it will already have gained some familiarity from the journey), tipped on its side so the patient can get in and out as it wishes, and provide food and water. Artificial heat is not necessary and if the open end of the box faces away from any major source of draught, is close to a wall allowing just enough space for the patient to get in and out, and the box is filled with hay, this will provide sufficient comfort.

Food

As indicated earlier, the badger is not hard to please so far as food is concerned and being shut in does not appear to adversely affect their appetites. Virtually any kind of meat will be acceptable, with tinned dog or cat meat as the cheapest and easiest to provide. In fact a large tin of dog meat mixed with dog biscuit, together with a bowl of water, will provide a perfectly satisfactory diet for the duration of the patient's stay, although it will also very much appreciate an occasional raw egg (left in the shell), a dead day-old chick or two if you can get them, or any dead mammal or bird you may come across if it has obviously been killed in a road accident. If you haven't anything else initially, a bowl of bread and milk will go down well.

Force-feeding

Attempting to force-feed an adult badger is fraught with danger and is most definitely not recommended.

Symptoms, Diagnosis and Treatment

Injuries. Badgers are very often the victims of road accidents, and suffer wide-ranging injuries. They are also frequently caught in snares, and one researcher told us that a badger he had been tracking with a radio collar around its neck, actually got caught in a snare three times during one night. It would seem that it is their insular attitude to life rather than any lack of intelligence that accounts for this.

More often than not the badger is killed when hit by a car. Because of its size it presents a serious problem to the driver, and if the car is travelling at speed, it may veer off the road and a serious accident result. Occasionally, however, crash injuries are not fatal. Unless injuries are slight (in which case the badger will disappear and not come to the attention of the public), the animal may be found in a dazed or shocked condition at the side of or near the road.

Badgers are very tough and although the injuries may look severe it is well worth taking the animal to a veterinary surgeon for examination and possible treatment. Broken legs can be set and lacerations cleaned and sutured. In most cases it will be necessary to anaesthetize the animal for even the simplest treatment, but nowadays this presents no real difficulty to the veterinary surgeon.

One of the reasons that badgers so often get knocked down by cars is that in their night-time explorations and food hunts, they usually follow well-defined paths – easily visible to us in daytime – which they have trodden out over many decades of use. When a road (even a motorway) is built across one of these ancient tracks the badgers will continue to use it and amble across the road oblivious to the traffic.

Because of concern for the number of casualties in a species that in the whole of Britain probably numbers no more than fifty to a hundred thousand – and concern for the motorist also – an underpass was made on the M1 involving a stream culvert which was reasonably close to the badger path. The sides of the main road were fenced to force the badgers to change their route and use the culvert when crossing the road. Materials were paid for by the road construction unit and all the work was done by volunteers. The project was successful and the badgers now use this detour regularly. Subsequently, in 1973, a similar structure was built under the M53 motorway in Cheshire, and later under the M5 motorway in Somerset. Since then some others have been built and the principle established to the benefit of both motorist and badger.

Diseases and Poisoning. Badgers are susceptible to a number of diseases, but except for one – tuberculosis – it is most unlikely that the public will come across a diseased badger that might need care and attention. The badger unfortunately seems to be highly susceptible to the bovine type of tuberculosis. This disease not only affects the internal organs, in particular the kidneys and digestive system, but also causes suppurating sores from fight wounds. As with most wild animals the symptoms are hidden, or do not become obvious until it is well advanced. According to reports, the disease seems to alter the behaviour pattern of the badger, and it is often found wandering about alone in the daytime – a relatively unusual occurrence.

Should you come across a badger that has no apparent injury, yet it is disinclined to move when approached – a careful note should be made of the spot, and the police or a representative of the Ministry of Agriculture should be informed. If a dead badger be found it is best to make a careful note of the site and to inform the police or local authority because it may have tuberculosis.

To guard against the possible unwitting spread of tuberculosis, translocation of badgers from one area to another should not be carried out without first consulting the Ministry of Agriculture's veterinary department for that area. There is circumstantial evidence that badgers may be responsible for spreading the disease to cattle, and for this reason the Ministry of Agriculture has authorized the gassing of badger setts in those areas by full-time pest-control officers after consultation with their veterinary department. This means of course that many healthy, non-affected badgers are killed, for even in the worst areas the incidence of infected badgers was never higher than 20 per cent. However, because no satisfactory test exists for determining whether or not a live badger is suffering from tuberculosis, the Ministry of Agriculture feel it necessary to carry out this extermination policy. Up to date, in excess of 10,000 setts have been gassed, killing an unknown number of badgers, for once gassed the setts are sealed. However on a rough estimate of three badgers per sett, bearing in mind that many setts contain more badgers than three whereas other setts may be empty, 30,000 out of a total of between 50–100,000 may have been exterminated.

Fortunately the badgers are still breeding fairly prolifically, and as yet there is no indication that the species is endangered. But it is most important to emphasize that these measures are carried out by Ministry of Agriculture officials in charge of the control of tuberculosis in cattle. *Under no circumstances* should farmers take the matter into their own hands and start exterminating badgers. The Ministry officials know exactly where the risks are, and have informed the farmers in those areas. Outside those areas there is absolutely no risk to cattle, nor of course to the public.

General Care

An outside pen for a wild adult badger is not an easy or cheap item to provide. Like the fox (Chapter 14), the badger is good at both climbing and digging. In climbing ability fox and badger are probably well matched but in digging, the badger is undoubtedly superior, and while the general principles of the pen described in Chapter 14 would apply for the badger, one or two modifications would be advisable for complete security.

In the early stages of being incarcerated in the pen, a badger is apt to bite and worry at the wire itself, even making its mouth bleed. A fence of only 16 gauge may not break, but it would certainly become very distorted by this attention, and 12 or even 10 gauge is recommended. The ground wire in a badger pen should be placed some distance underground, allowing the animal to do a certain amount of digging. The wire should cover the whole of the pen area as the badger may commence excavations at any point, very often under its sleeping quarters, and depending on the nature of the ground, can make quite an appreciable length of tunnel in one night. Just how far underground the base wire is placed depends entirely on how much you yourself want to do or have done. About 12–18in. (30–45cm) would be fine.

If you can provide a sleeping box which can be closed (e.g. a channel for a sliding door see Fig. 15), this will help very considerably when the time comes for release. By this time your badger won't be at all easy to catch or handle.

Release

All being well, the badger should be asleep in its box when you slide the door into place. Without pain to either side, badger and box can both be transported to the point of release – preferably as near as possible to the point where it was found, enabling the animal to return to its home sett. If the release is made at dusk, the sliding door can be removed and the animal tipped out unceremoniously. It won't protest at this undignified exit, and will almost certainly lope off immediately in the direction of home.

If it is impossible for some reason to return the animal to its home ground, it is preferable to effect the release in an area free of active badger setts, rather than in some other badgers' area. Your local County Naturalists' Trust should be able to assist in selecting a suitable spot.

Orphans

It is an exceptional circumstance that will bring in cubs less than about six weeks old, as this is the very youngest they are likely to be above ground of their own accord. Even then, they are unlikely to move far from the sett entrance where they can bolt back underground at the first hint of disturbance. If a cub should be found on its own, the chances are it will be over three months old, in which case it should be able to feed itself.

On one or two occasions we have had younger cubs brought in, and once three arrived, having been dug out purely by accident, which were no more than two weeks old. These were reared in the same manner and on the same mixture as for fox cubs (see Chapter 14), but a baby's bottle with a premature baby's teat was used instead of the syringe. Bottle feeding continued until the cubs were just over three months old (thirteen weeks in fact), but we reduced it in the latter stages, with only two bottle feeds a day in the final week.

Two of these cubs were sows, and the boar we lost very early on in the proceedings. He was constantly being sucked on a sensitive part of his anatomy by the other two, in spite of regular feeds, until he became quite sore. We ought to have separated them but didn't think to do so. Whether this was a contributing factor in his death is difficult to ascertain, but should we be presented with a similar situation in the future, we would certainly separate differently sexed youngsters.

A move outside can be made before the end of weaning (at about 8 or 9 weeks) into a pen as described for adult casualties. A portable sett should again be provided, unless the cubs can be released directly from the pen into a suitable locality, in which case a burrow more resembling a natural sett can be provided. If the cubs cannot be so released, a good deal of thought must go into just where they are placed, seeking all possible advice and not releasing too early (about five months minimum). They must be strong enough and large enough to have a reasonable chance with any possible adversary they might encounter. With the permission of the owner, it might be possible to construct an artificial sett in a piece of woodland not already occupied by badgers, which would help very much in giving them a good start. Of course there is no guarantee they would stay there but *any* release to the wild of a hand-reared youngster is a risk. As someone once said in a different context, 'if you put up too many fences against the risks, you end by shutting out life itself'.

Hand-reared badger cubs make an easier transition than many from a sheltered existence to a wild one, and the change to a nocturnal way of life seems quite effortless and can happen suddenly. One day they will be pottering about in broad daylight and then, just as though a switch had been thrown, they may never be seen again during the day. We recall one particular young sow called Hazel, one of three brought in at about three months old. The boar and sow had been found dead on a road, and the three youngsters were found on the verge nearby. It was some time before they were brought to us, and one was very weak on arrival and died overnight. A second went to another home leaving Hazel who was bottle fed for a week or so before she would deign to feed herself. We allowed her the freedom of the premises and when she began to get out and about, a friendship was struck with a lamb which had also been hand-reared. They used to spend all day together nosing around, or having a rough and tumble. It was quite hilarious to watch Hazel taking a sudden nip at the lamb's foot then setting off as fast as she could go with the lamb bouncing along like a rubber ball behind her.

After a time, the lamb was transferred elsewhere leaving Hazel to potter about on her own, and during one particular day's explorations, she found her way under a large shed. She stayed there for quite a time and when she finally emerged, it was to spend the rest of the day carrying her bedding from where she had been living to her new home under the shed. We watched these operations with interest and the furniture removal was completed by about mid-afternoon, at which time Hazel disappeared under the shed and was never again seen in daylight. She lived there for quite some time before finally making her way into the countryside where we hope she survived. From reports received subsequently, we know she was still living a year afterwards.

Badger

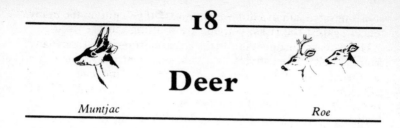

18

Deer

Muntjac   *Roe*

These are our largest wild animals, and the largest of the group, the red deer, stands about 4ft 6in. (1.35 metres) to the top of the head. With full antlers, this can be over 6ft (1.8 metres). There are now six species of deer living wild in Britain, although none of them cover the whole country. In descending order of size they are the red, the fallow, the sika, the roe, with the muntjac and the Chinese water deer the smallest, both about 2ft (60cm) tall.

Most people can make a correct identification of a deer, although they may not be able to put a name to the particular species. They will experience most difficulty with the muntjac, which is a somewhat strange-looking animal, and the Chinese water deer, which has tusks instead of antlers.

Probably the best known, and arguably the most attractive of the group, is the fallow with its spotted coat (usually) and elegant palmated (flat) antlers. It is familiar because many herds are kept in city parks and the parks of a good many stately (and not so stately) homes, where they can be seen grazing in broad daylight. Its wild counterpart is chiefly nocturnal and/or very shy and secretive, and who can blame them when they are pursued either by poachers or by vandals on horseback with packs of dogs?

There are now quite extensive moves afoot to 'farm' red deer and if meat is to be eaten, this practice might well bring down the price of venison and make poaching an uneconomic proposition – a much surer way of bringing it to an end than any possible preventative measures. It is too early, at the time of writing, to make a reasoned judgement on the subject of deer farming except to say, like every other man/animal relationship, that it will undoubtedly lead to at least *some* abuses of the animal in the name of a quick profit. Already one deplorable but very lucrative practice has crept into the deer-farming scene (notably in New Zealand), which is the 'harvesting' of velvet (the covering of skin on the antlers while they are growing each year). This is sold for high prices, principally in the Far East, as an aphrodisiac. Apart from other considerations, the mere fact that the animal needs an anaesthetic each time the operation is carried out is sufficient to condemn it (see *Symptoms, Diagnosis and Treatment*).

Possible Handling Hazards

The handling of deer by inexperienced people alone, particularly the larger species, is not recommended. Even the little roe is a powerful and potentially dangerous animal which has been known to kill a man. The trouble is that most people are apt to be imbued with the gentle and delicate 'Bambi' image of deer, whereas the hoof of a red deer can disembowel, and we have seen severe facial lacerations, almost removing an eye, caused by a fallow deer on only three legs.

In most areas where deer are present, there is someone with experience who will attend to a casualty, and the local police or RSPCA Inspector will doubtless know where he or she is to be found. We most strongly urge you to call upon such a person when an injured deer is encountered. The following notes are intended more for information, and should only be acted upon if there is absolutely *no* help available or forthcoming.

Approach and Capture

If the deer is on its feet, it will probably run away when approached, although a male *may* launch an attack, particularly during the rutting season (in the autumn). In a confined situation, *any* deer may try to fend off what it considers to be an attack. With the female, this will take the form of rearing on her hind legs and 'boxing' with her front hooves, while a male will usually attack with the head, whether equipped with antlers or not. In such a situation, tranquillization by darting may well be called for and this is most definitely a job for the expert (see *Symptoms, Diagnosis and Treatment*). Deer do not bite.

If the animal is lying down, try to keep the head on the ground, cushioning it with a coat, but keep well clear of the hooves until it is time for the move.

Transportation

Before moving the patient, it may be desirable to 'hobble' it – to tie its legs loosely together to prevent it rising – and again we must reiterate the warning, do not underestimate the strength of what appear to be slender delicate legs, or you may lose an eye. In the case of a male, the antlers will have to be protected or, in some cases, removed by an expert. In the case of a pricket (second-year male), when there is simply a 'spike' with no tines (branching spikes), a piece of hosepipe can be slipped over each or a piece of sacking tied round each. In the case of a mature male in velvet, no attempt should be made to remove the antlers, but they must be protected with lots of padding on each (with wooden splints on each antler), and *between* the antlers. At other times the antlers are in effect dead, and no pain or adverse effect is caused by removing them. The cut is best made above the brow tine (the first spike which sticks out to the front) using an embryotomy wire, for preference, which any veterinary surgeon will have among his equipment (although a saw can be used).

A minimum floor area in the vehicle of about 2 × 4ft (60 × 120cm) will be required to transport a red deer, and it may require four people to lift the animal.

Initial Care

In our experience, wild adult deer do not like to be inside a building. They appear to suffer quite severely from claustrophobia, and this may be a contributing factor to the death of a casualty so kept. An open paddock with plenty of undergrowth or a few bales of straw to screen the animal from view is preferable. In the case of a patient which cannot move, some kind of awning should be rigged to protect it from heavy rain (which it will be unable to shake off), or it should be placed under a tree with plenty of foliage which will serve the same purpose. Some water should be administered and this can be done quite easily, dribbling it into the mouth with the aid of a plastic syringe, and giving a generous quantity – up to half a pint (300ml) for a red. Of course if the animal will drink by itself there is no need for administration, but an initial intake of liquid, one way or the other, will undoubtedly be beneficial. A bowl of water should also be left within easy reach, and some food provided.

Food

If you can get hold of some, ivy will tempt the appetite of most deer. Rose petals also seem to be most palatable, and other suitable foods include the leaves of broad-leafed trees, grass, hay, root and leaf vegetables, nut kernels, chick pellets, cereals, and one red deer of our acquaintance is very fond of pilchards in tomato sauce!

In general, a deer casualty's willingness to take nourishment is a good pointer to the severity of its injury. In other words, if it refuses to feed voluntarily, its chances of ultimate recovery are rather slim.

Force-feeding

Force-feeding is a fairly easy task and can be undertaken if it is thought desirable. But do always bear in mind the dangers as outlined previously. A plastic syringe can be used although it will need to be filled a good many times at each feed in order to give sufficient nourishment, particularly to the larger species who will require at least 1 pint (600ml) two or three times a day. An empty washing-up liquid bottle can be used and the food can be squeezed into the side of the mouth direct from this. Use Lactol and/or a baby cereal at the thickest it will come out of the container and do not rush it, allow the animal plenty of time to swallow the mixture.

Symptoms, Diagnosis and Treatment

Injuries. As with badgers, deer are frequently victims of road accidents, with broken legs or dislocated limbs as the principal injuries, together with abrasions and lacerations of the skin. This applies primarily to fallow and roe deer in this country. Occasionally they get caught in snares, and one recent sufferer we saw had to be shot. The snare had tightened around the animal's neck and must have finally broken it after lacerating the skin. It had occurred several weeks earlier for the skin was beginning to grow over the wire as it encircled the neck. The windpipe had been partly severed and the animal was breathing through the hole in its neck as well as through its mouth. This obviously greatly impaired its ability to get about, and it was seen to be trailing behind the family group, often standing on its own. For this reason it was singled out and caught, and the snare – not visible from a distance because of the skin growing over it – was found and the animal shot. The injuries were so severe that it would have caused a considerable amount of suffering to have attempted to treat the animal. A quite horrific example of man's inhumanity to animal.

It is not uncommon to find deer trapped in wire fencing (apart from wire snares). The animal may have attempted to jump over or through the fence and got stuck. Sometimes the wire breaks and a portion remains wrapped round a leg.

The wisest course of action is to mark the spot carefully and seek help as quickly as possible. Deer are easily frightened, especially when caught in wire, and may cause themselves much more serious injuries when approached. If the animal is exhausted it may be approached slowly and carefully and then held firmly while the wire is cut away. Otherwise it should be darted with a tranquillizer and this means the assistance of a veterinary surgeon. The tranquillizer used is a powerful drug called Etorphine (M99), that has an antidote. The dart must be loaded with the correct dose according to the weight of the animal and fired into the muscle (usually the rump). It is absorbed and acts within 10–15 minutes. After being hit, the animal runs away, slows down gradually, staggers, and falls. It can then be secured and given the antidote.

Occasionally in certain areas, deer have been found with heads of arrows from crossbows sticking in them. The animal has to be caught, tranquillized, and the arrowhead removed – which of course requires the services of a veterinary surgeon. Gunshot wounds from poachers are not uncommon, and again help should be sought to catch and treat the animal.

Perruque head (from the French, meaning a wig) is the abnormal grotesque growth of velvet antler as a result of damage to the testicles either by injury or castration. This stops the production of the sex hormone, testosterone, which controls the antler growth cycle. This abnormal growth is seen in roe deer where there is some additional new growth each summer adding to the antler growth which is never shed. Because it remains in velvet the growth is liable to damage and haemorrhage, for the velvet covering the growth is really skin amply supplied with blood vessels.

If a young deer under nine months of age is castrated, the pedicle from which the antler normally grows, never forms and the deer will never grow antlers throughout its life. If castration or severe damage occurs to an adult stag whilst in velvet (as the antlers are growing) growth continues for a while and finally ceases. If castration or severe damage occurs to an adult stag with hard antlers they are immediately shed (within three weeks) and growth commences at once. But the antlers never reach their proper size and shape, though they grow for a longer time, and they remain in velvet and never harden.

Diseases and Poisoning. Deer usually appear fairly healthy, but this is not uncommon with wild animals. In spite of this, they suffer from a variety of diseases including tuberculosis, foot and mouth disease, cancers and both internal and external parasites.

In the wild when an animal becomes diseased or old and debilitated it falls easy prey to predators. This may seem cruel, but it terminates quickly, although traumatically, an otherwise lengthy period of suffering. Prey animals must show no signs of weakness to predators lest they be singled out, and for this reason, disease is often fairly advanced before the animal allows the symptoms to show. It is therefore possible that members of the public, while walking in the countryside, may come across a deer that is disinclined to move, perhaps unsteady on its feet, and looks thin (though often a heavy coat hides the real condition of the animal). Emaciation causes wasting of the facial muscles and a depletion of the fat behind and around the eye. This causes the eye to sink in the socket, which is immediately obvious. Such cases should be reported to the owner of the land who may claim ownership of the deer, or the RSPCA if there is a problem. The cause could be any one of those mentioned above, and an examination by a veterinary surgeon is required.

General Care

If a deer is to be kept for any length of time, it must have a paddock of adequate size so that the area does not become totally contaminated with droppings, which is a hazard to the animal's health. To house a single red deer on a long-term basis, we would recommend an area not less than 50 × 25 yards (45 × 22.5 metres) and about half this for a roe. The paddock should be enclosed by a 6-foot (1.8 metres) high fence which can be of sheep netting and should include some shelter from wind, which deer do not seem to like very much, and sun. Shelter from rain and other elements is not necessary for a fit or reasonably fit animal, but is for an immobile patient (see page 149). Bear in mind that any trees, shrubs or plants within the boundary are likely to suffer grievous bodily harm!

Do not expect the natural contents of the paddock to sustain the deer but continue to provide food from the list given. We generally give a type of cattle mix usually called 'dairy mixture', some chick pellets, and peanut kernels as a regular diet, supplemented with other titbits from time to time.

Orphans

A good many deer picked up as orphans are not really orphans at all. This is particularly true of the roe who will leave her youngster/s hiding in the grass while she grazes in the vicinity. The kid/s will not move at any approach, and of course they are found apparently alone and 'lost' when the mother will, in fact, be watching from somewhere very close by. Anyone needing reassurance on this point should note the spot where they have seen the youngster and leave without touching it at all, returning an hour or so later to see if it is still there. The chances are it won't be. But if it is then there *is* some reason to wonder, particularly if the youngster is by this time making peeping noises indicating distress.

There are, of course, many circumstances producing quite genuine orphans, such as poachers killing the mother or, as in a recent case we had, the mother being killed by a vehicle, leaving twin kids sitting dutifully by her dead body, waiting for her to show them what to do next. In these circumstances, the youngsters must obviously be taken into care but more often than not, this will change the whole course of their lives. It is most difficult to keep a young deer from becoming imprinted on the person feeding it and to lose its fear of other humans – a fatal affliction for any wild animal.

If more than one arrive at the same time, there is a better chance of a 'wild rearing'. The roe, for instance, normally has twins, and the Chinese water deer will produce four or five or even more. We have reared a number of pairs and been able to release them to the wild, whereas most hand-reared single deer have to go to some sheltered environment.

Incidentally, young deer are variously called calf, fawn or kid, depending on their species, just as some adults are called stag and hind and others buck and doe.

Unlike adult casualties, it is safe and indeed desirable to keep the youngsters indoors for a time, at least until they are well accustomed to accepting the bottle from you. If placed out of doors from the start, they will simply tear around in a blind panic at your approach.

We always use Lactol for feeding young deer although there are several other products on the market for human babies which have a very similar content and do not carry the dreaded VAT. Whatever you use stick with it for the duration of the weaning otherwise you will most certainly encounter problems when trying to change over, not least of which may be flat rejection of the new food. Ordinary cows' milk is not suitable.

A maximum of five feeds per day is sufficient for even the very youngest, but the actual quantity will vary considerably, depending on the species. A roe, for instance will start at about 5 fl. oz. (150ml) and a red at about 15 fl. oz. (450ml), and these quantities should be increased as the youngster manages to empty the bottle easily. You cannot overfeed as the infant will simply stop sucking when it has had enough, but time must be allowed during a feed for the odd scamper about.

An ordinary baby's feeding bottle is fine for deer up to roe size but for the larger species, needing more than 8 fl. oz. (284ml) at a 'sitting', an ordinary pint (568ml) lemonade bottle or similar can be used with a calf teat attached.

We have frequently found that young deer taken out for a short stroll following a feed will eat a bit of soil. Whether this is of any great significance is hard to say but we now always keep a bowl of soil in the pen so that they can help themselves should they so wish. A selection of solid food should also be offered from an early stage. Although the youngsters will not be able to make much of a showing, they like to try nibbling at various items.

Milk feeds will need to continue until at least mid-September although when the change can be made from drinking out of a bottle to out of a bowl or bucket is an individual matter, not even one of species. We have had some (of various species) drinking from a bowl or bucket as early as June, and some that would not even try until late July.

There is equally no hard and fast rule for the move out of doors. As indicated earlier, we make this move as soon as the youngsters have an established feeding pattern and no longer shy away when their 'foster-mum' comes to feed them. In this respect, it is by far the best if one person undertakes the whole of the bottle feeding.

A paddock as described for adult casualties should be provided with the added refinement of an open fronted box of sufficient size for the species (and numbers) concerned, furnished with straw for bedding. Young deer will usually use such a sleeping box if provided, but if they simply bed down under a bush, don't worry about it.

If they haven't finished drinking milk by mid-September, start diluting the feeds (which should be no more than one a day by this time) until they are simply water and the youngster gets the message.

Release may present a great problem as indicated earlier. If the youngster is so tame that it has completely lost its natural timidity, the chances are that it will walk up to the first person who comes along. That person might be the wrong one, and the fruits of your labour might be knocked on the head and wind up in a deep freeze. If you have been skilful (or lucky) and the animal runs away when approached – at least from other people – then by all means try a release in an area already frequented by the particular species. If it shows *no* fear, then the only course is to find a home for it in some private park. Your local County Naturalists' Trust or RSPCA Inspector may have some suggestions to offer, and the British Deer Society may be able to help place the animal.

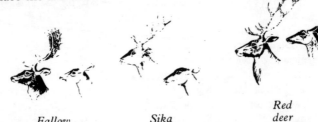

Fallow

Sika

Red deer

PART THREE
OTHER WILDLIFE

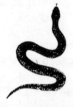

Adder

*Sand
lizard*

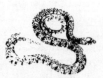

*Grass
snake*

*Smooth
snake*

19

Snakes & Lizards

Very few people will ever have the opportunity of giving assistance to the sick and injured creatures covered in this and the following two chapters. But if ill-treatment is prevented their inclusion in this book will have been justified.

There are only a few species of snakes native to the British Isles and they are rarely seen by the public. Even so they usually evoke fear in spite of the fact that only one, the adder, is poisonous.

Snakes are cold blooded. This does not mean that their blood is cold – indeed if it were, the animals would be comatose or at least very lethargic – but that they are unable to produce enough body heat by metabolic processes and control their temperature as accurately as mammals do. They rely instead on the sun to warm them into activity, and they must hibernate in the winter months.

They have an outer skin of scales and no skin glands so that, contrary to popular belief, snakes are dry to the touch. They cannot sweat for, apart from having no skin glands, they have an outer layer of transparent skin over the top of the scales. This covers even their eyes, so that tears have to escape through the nostrils.

None of the three species of snakes in Britain have any vestige of limbs. On average they have 150 vertebrae, each carrying two ribs all the way to the vent with no breastbone, and then a further 50 vertebrae without ribs in the tail. Their teeth are not in their jaws but in a number of bars running lengthways in the mouth. They have neither eyelids nor ears and so are deaf to sound, but are highly sensitive to vibrations. The tongue is the sensitive organ of touch.

Our only poisonous snake, the adder, has a short thick body, almost 3 feet (90cm) long. The sexes differ in colour and size, and indeed there is quite a variation in colour between individuals of the same sex. But all have a central zig-zag dark line down the centre of the back, and an inverted V on top of the head, although on darker-coloured snakes this is hard to see. They have two large poison fangs which they will only use if surprised or cornered. Nevertheless it is not uncommon to see young cattle with a very much thickened leg, at least as far up as the knee and sometimes higher, caused by a bite from an adder. It looks much more serious than it is, as the animal does not seem to be in very much pain, and the swelling goes down in due course.

Adders are nocturnal and bask in the sun during the day. They feed principally on small mammals but will also take small reptiles, amphibia and insect larvae. They drink water, so it is important if you have one captive for treatment that you give it water to drink (it will not eat in captivity). The young snakes are born alive in August after a gestation of four months. From mid October until April two or three will hibernate together in a hollow under a tree stump or under heaps of stones and in the heather. The adder's chief enemies are man, hedgehogs, poultry, goats and cats.

The British grass snake is larger – 3–4 feet (90–120cm) long – and seems to grow throughout its life. It is an olive grey brown or dark green in colour and lays twelve to fifty eggs in July or August in rich mould or manure heaps where they incubate for six to eight weeks. The baby snake inside has a small tooth to help it break out of the shell, which quickly drops away after hatching.

The grass snake is largely aquatic. Unlike the adder, the grass snake soon becomes tame and quite responsive to its human keeper. However, when first caught, and therefore stressed and frightened, it will void at both ends a stinking excreta which has a revolting garlic-like smell. As they do not bite, this is its only protection.

The smooth snake which is generally – but rarely – found in the south of England, is rather similar at first sight to the grass snake, but is smaller and usually darker. It is listed on the schedule of protected animals.

Britain has three native lizards and one of them, the sand lizard, is endangered. As the name implies it lives in sandy soils, and is larger than the common lizard. Both have four limbs each with five toes. The common lizard, which has a regular territory, lives on heather-clad hillsides. Lizards hibernate from October to April, several together in deep holes which they have dug. Six to twelve eggs are laid in July and August and hatch almost at once. Care must be taken in handling lizards for their tails are brittle and easily break off and they do not properly re-grow.

The same applies to the third species of British lizard, the slow worm, which normally has a finely tapered tail but is often seen with a fairly stumpy one indicating that at some time or other the tail has been broken off and not properly reformed. To the layman the slow worm looks exactly like a snake. But it really is a legless lizard up to 16 or 17in. (42–42.5cm) long. It can be readily distinguished because it has eyelids like lizards and teeth around the borders of the jaw. It is semi-nocturnal, coming out to feed in the late afternoon and evening, and is a great friend of the gardener for it has a good appetite for slugs, snails and various insects and earthworms. Indeed no garden should be without a pair.

Possible Handling Hazards

Adders are poisonous and when frightened they will bite. On the front of the upper jaw are two large fangs which lie flat when the mouth is closed, but which are pushed perpendicular by the opening of the mouth. At the same time the gland containing the poison is squeezed, causing it to flow down the hollow teeth. The poison is in fact a saliva which digests the prey as well as paralyzing it.

When free in the wild the adder or viper is not aggressive, and its natural instinct is to seek cover. But when caught or cornered it will try to bite. However, its jaws do not normally open wide enough to bite the legs of adults, and it is usually fingers or toes or limbs of children that get bitten. Few cases are reported in Britain and there are very few deaths. One anti-serum is available at some hospitals, but it is not essential. The best treatment is to open the wound to encourage bleeding and suck out the poison. A tourniquet may be applied above the wound before this is done and loosened every 5–10 minutes. Keep the person quiet and reassured.

The grass snake can bite, but is not poisonous.

Lizards and slow worms are quite harmless.

Approach and Capture

No attempts should be made to approach and capture an animal of this group unless it is obviously injured and can be helped, or alternatively it has to be moved for its own safety or that of human beings.

The simplest way to catch a snake or lizard is with a catching net (see Fig. 1). Once in the net it can be transferred to a cotton bag.

Transportation

The snake or lizard can be carried in a cotton bag which can be placed in a box if necessary.

Initial Care

Rest and quiet in a covered ventilated box with sand on the floor, a temperature of 22–25 C (71–77 F), and drinking water are the important points. They will not usually feed in this initial stage of their captivity.

Food

The grass snake will soon become tame and may take food – a small freshly killed mouse, dead day-old chick, or insect larvae. However, they do not eat regularly in the wild, gorging themselves when they do. Adders are more nervous and very, very rarely feed in captivity. This only becomes important if they are captive for more than a few weeks (they can go without food for 2 to 3 months), see below.

Symptoms, Diagnosis and Treatment

Like all other animals, reptiles can be injured and suffer from disease. Injuries can be accidental such as being run over by a car or stepped on by an animal. They should be humanely put to sleep if the injuries seem extensive. But remember that the slow worm and the other lizards can and do lose their tails without suffering even shock in the process. Snakes, on the other hand, do not have brittle tails and injuries should be treated. If the wound is kept clean it will generally heal fairly rapidly. Snakes and reptiles will generally feed in captivity, but the adder will not, and if treatment is prolonged it may have to be force-fed by simply putting a dead day-old chick or mouse down its throat with forceps. Squeezing the sides of the jaws will open the mouth.

It is extremely difficult for the expert and impossible for the layman to diagnose disease in reptiles. They show no consistent recognizable symptoms except loss of weight or diarrhoea and diagnosis must usually be made on post-mortem examination. Even if the reptile looks ill, leave it alone.

General Care

The aim must be to cure the animal as quickly as possible. Once a wound is healing well the snake can be safely released. Any kind of smooth sided box or an empty aquarium with sand on the bottom will serve for convalescence. Keep in a fairly warm room (about 25 C, 77 F) with water always available.

Release

It is best to release the snake where it was found if possible, for it will know the area, and has more chance of survival.

20

Amphibia

Amphibia are more primitive creatures than reptiles. Frogs and toads have nine vertebrae but no ribs, and a three-chambered heart. In spite of the fact that their skin is smooth and moist and contains a great number of glands, they do not produce the same nervousness in human beings that snakes or even lizards do. They have glands in the skin containing different pigments which can be squeezed to drive the colour to the surface thus enabling the animal to match its colour to its surroundings. They have many predators and this is one of their major protective mechanisms. The toad has another, not shared by common frogs or newts, in that its skin is covered with glands that give out an irritant poison when roughly handled. This poison will not penetrate the human skin, but will irritate the mucous lining of the mouth and eye. No dog that has ever picked up a toad will do so again. He will quickly drop it and will go off shaking his head and working his tongue to get rid of the irritation.

With neither ribs nor diaphragm, breathing is done by the throat. The frog or toad closes its mouth and nostrils and forces air down into the lungs. It does this at quite a fast rate but if you look carefully you can see the underneath part of the throat pulsating. During hibernation in winter, oxygen is absorbed through the pores all over the skin and mouth so that breathing as such is unnecessary.

There are two species of toad native to Britain, the common toad as its name implies is the one usually seen, and the natterjack toad which is endangered. The common toad is also a friend of the gardener for it has an insatiable appetite for slugs, caterpillars, beetles and other insects. Like reptiles they shed their skin every few weeks as they grow. The skin splits down the back and gradually peels off which they help along with their hands and feet. Toads move slowly with a sort of crawl or short heavy hops – in fact everything about them is slow except their large, flat, sticky, elastic tongues which can be flicked out rapidly for about 2in. (5cm) to catch their prey.

Toads hibernate in deep dry holes far from water during the

months of October to March. They then head for ponds to mate and attract each other with croaking and whining bleats. They embrace for a week or more and the female produces between 2,000–7,000 eggs in two parallel strings from 10–15 feet (3–4.5 metres) long which trail around the water weeds in the pond. The eggs hatch into tadpoles which reach their maximum size in seventy days. After a further fifteen days, a minute toad emerges and heads for the shore. Many are taken by predators and the lucky ones take five years to reach maturity.

The natterjack toad is smaller with a much smoother skin, a golden line on the back and a green iris. The skin poison it exudes has an odd smell rather like india rubber. They neither hop nor crawl and in fact have been called the running toad. The natterjack is an endangered species and is protected by law in Britain. It is found in isolated populations.

The common or grass frog is the only native British frog. It is longer and slimmer than the toads with no warts and no poison. The skin is smooth and moist and not unpleasant to touch. Unfortunately, it has countless enemies – including man, who uses it for experimental and teaching purposes. And in spite of the fact that it lays thousands of eggs, numbers have been seriously declining.

Newts are much smaller than toads or frogs, and we have three species in Britain which live for the most part on land except during the breeding season. They are not often seen because of their nocturnal habits. They too feed on insects.

They differ from frogs by having fourteen to seventeen pairs of ribs and a tail that is flattened from side to side. The eggs are laid one by one rolled in the leaf of a plant and hatch in about thirteen days to a larval form with an almost transparent body.

Handling Hazards
The only problem is with the toad. Its irritant secretions will not normally penetrate the skin, but they could hurt if you have an open cut on your hand.

Capture
As for reptiles.

Transportation
Transportation should be in moist surroundings i.e. damp moss or tissues in a wooden box.

Initial Care
Keep quiet and moist in an old aquarium in which there is some water and a dry standing area.

Food
Slugs and insects.

Symptoms, Diagnosis and Treatment
The authors have only experience of injuries and they usually heal fairly well. If a limb of a newt gets damaged it can regrow from a stump.

Release
Release should be in the place or area where the animal was found.

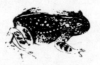

Natterjack toad

Common frog

Male palmate newt

Male common newt

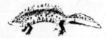

Male crested newt

21

Fish

Fish are also cold blooded, and have an advantage over reptiles and amphibia in that the temperature and often the composition of their environment only varies within narrow limits. They have become so specialized that freshwater fish will not, as a rule, live in the sea, nor sea fish in rivers and lakes. There are exceptions, and the salmon is the most obvious. However it does spend most of its life in the sea, and on entering rivers to mate and spawn, its physiology changes drastically and eventually it dies there.

Because the body fluids of river fish are more salty than river water there is a tendency for water to be absorbed; so the fish does not drink and it passes urine. The body fluids of a sea fish are less salty than the sea and there is a tendency for it to lose fluids; so it drinks and it does not pass urine.

Like all animals fish require oxygen and must eliminate carbon dioxide, a product of metabolism. This is accomplished by the gills which act as a sort of lung. The oxygen in the water is partly dissolved from the air and partly given off by plants in the daytime when photosynthesis occurs. The colder the water the more oxygen there is present. And of course the greater the surface exposed to the air as in rapids or in a waterfall, the more oxygen is dissolved. So slow-moving rivers or still lakes in summer will provide less oxygen for fish and there will be still less should there be black, smelly, decaying matter along the banks and bottom – all of which means fewer fish.

Another advantage of water is that it supports the body weight, and so, as one might expect, it is home to the largest animal that has ever lived – a mammal, not a fish – the blue whale. The largest fish is the whale shark which is not a whale, and certainly does not act like a shark, for it is a vegetarian. It grows to 50 feet (15 metres) in length.

As fish increase in size year by year their scales get bigger rather than become more numerous. And as growth is faster in the summer when food is more plentiful, each scale develops a ring for each year rather like trees. So it is possible to age the fish by counting these rings.

Some species of fish are loners and others such as cod live together in aggregations. Other species form schools where each individual is correctly spaced from the next, for swimming. And finally there are pods where the fish are so close as to be in actual physical contact.

Schooling is most common in pelagic (deep-sea) fish such as the herring. A big school behaves almost as if it were a single organism and the fish are usually of uniform size like 'cells'. These schools are prone to circle, playing 'follow my leader' especially in confined spaces. Sound may play a major part in keeping the school together, for not only do most fish have good 'hearing', but many make sounds, some of such low frequency as to be inaudible to the human ear. Scientists have recorded and played back these sounds and were able to make the school change direction. Watching a school gives one the impression that there is some central control mechanism, so perfectly do the individuals act together. However it could be that the human eye is unable to detect the minute movements of each individual beginning with the change of direction of one fish which then becomes the new leader.

Although fish are sensitive to sound, they cannot hear in our sense of the word, for they have no ears as we know them. They have neither ear drum nor inner ear structure which makes up the hearing apparatus in mammals. It seems likely that they sense sound waves using their gas bladder as a resonator. Certainly a fish can detect a footstep on the river bank and the beat of a ship's propeller.

Fish not only have most of the senses to which we are accustomed, but a further sense that records subtle changes in the flow of water around them. It is unique to fish and consists of a canal system called the lateral line that contains nerve organs connected to the brain. Scientists have yet to discover all the secrets of this 'sixth sense', but it seems to record disturbances in the water around the fish, and changes in the direction of flow, for cutting the nerves to the brain from these organs interrupts this ability. It is obviously valuable in keeping fish in schools at the correct distance from each other and telling fish where obstacles lie in murky water.

The sense of touch is carried by small nerve organs scattered over the skin and they are particularly abundant around the head and lips. The sense of smell is highly developed in most fish, which have the equivalent of our nostrils. Although they appear small, the cavity behind is lined with folded walls to provide a maximum surface for sensation. In most fish the sense of smell is so acute that they seem to use it rather than sight in seeking out their food. Sharks, for example, can smell blood from a great distance. It is thought to be this sense that guides the salmon thousands of miles back to the river of its birth to breed. And eels, another fish with a dramatic migratory cycle, are also said to use this sense of smell for navigation. It wasn't until the end of the eighteenth century that anyone had ever recorded a fresh-water eel with mature sex organs. In 1896 two Italian scientists found larval eels in the Straits of Messina. Then at the beginning of this century Danish scientists found that eels spawned in the Sargasso Sea at depths of about 200 fathoms and the larvae drifted with the Gulf Stream taking approximately two years to reach the coasts of Europe, by which time they are elvers about 3in. (7.5cm) long. They migrate up rivers in swarms and grow to yellow eels. Finally one summer they make for the sea, lose their digestive system, become silver in colour and migrate back to where they were born to breed and die.

Taste however is not well developed and few species have taste buds.

The eyes of fish function in much the same way as those of terrestrial mammals. There are of course some differences – for example, fish that feed on flies above the water have to compensate for refraction of light. There is also less light available in water, and so fish not only do without eyelids but they can manage with little or no contraction of the iris. Most of the time fish need only see a short distance ahead, and so vision is restricted, at best, to about 100 feet (30 metres). Since the lens is almost of the same density as water to allow for refraction, it has to be almost spherical. Because the eyes are set on either side of the head vision is monocular, and although this makes it difficult to judge distances it has the advantage of allowing the fish to see in more than one direction at a time. It is not known to what degree fish can see colour although it is generally accepted that all fish, except for sharks, have some colour vision.

The total fish harvest world wide has been climbing steadily, peaking at seventy million tons in 1970, and declining in the three years following. Experts believe it cannot be greater than a hundred million tons without upsetting the reproductive cycles. Most of this vast quantity of fish is caught in nets, hauled out of the sea and allowed to die on the decks and in the holds. Is it cruel? Do fish suffer? Can they feel pain?

This problem was investigated by a panel of experts under the chairmanship of Lord Cranbrook, himself a biologist, and their report was published in May 1980 after three years' work. They concluded that although there may be people who will argue that it cannot be proved beyond question that any vertebrate other than man feels pain, if any animals feel pain then the evidence suggests that all vertebrates (including fish) experience similar sensation to a greater or lesser degree.

Twenty-nine years earlier the government committee on Cruelty to Wild Animals said that pain was of the utmost value to animals in teaching the avoidance of what is harmful to it. 'Pain,' they say, 'is therefore a sensation of clear-cut biological usefulness . . .' But of course they were talking of what occurs in the wild, not the pain and suffering inflicted by man's sophisticated methods – to which animals are not biologically adapted.

Recent research has elucidated the nerve receptors and biochemical means of transmission of pain sensation. A polypeptide known as substance P is important in the transmission of pain, and a naturally occurring pain-killing substance which chemically resembles morphine and is called Enkephalin. Fish possess these chemicals at much the same levels as mammals, therefore when a fish is hooked it is kinder to kill it quickly before attempting to remove the hook. Thus it becomes a strange anomaly that though the Protection of Animals Act 1911 applies to all vertebrates including fish and reptiles, it is restricted to captive animals. A goldfish in a bowl is protected from unnecessary suffering but a goldfish in a river is not.

Fish are susceptible to a number of diseases and eight of these are notifiable to the authorities – most of them virus diseases which are not responsive to antibiotics. So even if you find and diagnose a diseased fish there is little that can be done apart from killing it as painlessly as possible (see Appendix B). It is also important to remember that apart from the fact that handling out of water with bare hands, or in a cloth, may be very painful, handling damages the skin, causing osmotic breakdown and rendering it more susceptible to infection. The stress may also precipitate disease. Skin infection, often fungal, is not uncommon after handling in an angling competition, for example, especially if the fish are kept in a crowded keep-net in a backwater where the flow of water is slow.

Information on the diseases of captive fish in fish farms or in tropical tanks is accumulating fast but it does not come within the scope of this book.

Fish can be easily poisoned. Nitrates from untreated sewage, chemical pollutants from factories, and run-off water from agricultural land treated with pesticides or herbicides, all take their toll on lake and river fish. The sea is large enough to dilute most poisons but occasionally disasters can occur. One of the worst is the red tide which can occur all over the world. When conditions are right a tiny dinoflagellate – a plankton – rapidly multiplies, and gives off a toxin which is poisonous to many species. In 1957 a Soviet research vessel reported sighting millions of dead fish floating in the Arabian Sea covering an area of 80,000 square miles (208,000 sq. km).

Fish have been found to have sub-lethal amounts of poisonous substances in their bodies without showing any symptoms of poisoning. But they are dangerous to eat, and poisonings of human beings have occurred, the most widely reported being of Japanese fisherfolk.

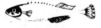

9-spined
stickleback

Trout

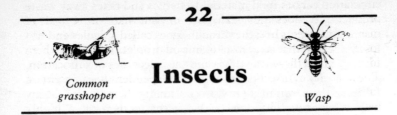

22

Common
grasshopper

Insects

Wasp

Insects cannot be ignored, and one good reason is the sheer number and diversity of them. One acre of forest soil probably contains 425 million insects, and the total population of insects on earth is estimated at about 10 billion billion. The total weight of all the insects on earth is about twelve times that of the human population. Their breeding rate is also astounding because they can produce dozens of generations per season. For example, the cabbage aphid will normally produce forty young per female and will have sixteen generations in a season. If all remained alive and bred, a single aphid at the beginning of the season would account for a total population of 1,560,000,000,000,000,000,000,000 by the end!

It is estimated that there are about five million species of living creatures on earth though only half have so far been identified, and 800,000 of these are insects. At least 20,000 are to be found in the United Kingdom.

What do we understand by the word insect? In biological terms insects all belong to the one phylum, or major subsection of the animal kingdom, called arthropoda, which means possessing jointed limbs and an external skeleton. Instead of having a skeleton like us surrounded by flesh, they have a hard, strengthened outer skeleton with the flesh or muscles and blood vessels and organs inside. Insects, in the biological sense that is, are the only arthropods to possess wings, and none of them have more than six true legs in the adult stage. The juvenile forms such as caterpillars, however, frequently have many more.

In this chapter we will use the word insect in its more colloquial sense to mean all those creepy crawlies that are obviously not fish, amphibia or reptiles. The biggest insects found in Britain today are the death's head hawk moth with a 5in. (12.5cm) wing span and the stag beetle which is 3in. (7.5cm) long. Large maybe, but small in comparison to the dragon-fly that lived in England three million years ago which had a 2 foot (60cm) wing span.

Insects do not have a respiratory system like us, their

circulation carries food material to tissues and takes away waste products. It does not transport oxygen like the blood of mammals. Insects breathe through tubes called spicules and it is for this reason that an aerosol of fine oil droplets is lethal to them for they block these tiny tubes and the insect dies of suffocation. The majority of insects live solitary, independent lives, intent on fulfilling their own needs and in continuing their species. Many have complicated life cycles that seem to demand a highly developed brain. But the behaviour is predetermined by genes. Some insects are truly social – for example, bees, wasps and ants – and behave almost as if they had no lives of their own, but were simply cells of the body which is the nest or hive.

Some insects are essentially parasitic on mammals and bite their host to obtain blood. Examples of this group are mosquitoes, midges, fleas, lice, bed bugs and horse flies. Quite a number of insects have stings which they will use for protection or defence. Others such as the ichneumon wasps use their sting to paralyze their prey.

Communication between insects is very important for most species and is accomplished in several ways. Moths use scent, called pheromone by scientists, which is emitted by the female and can be detected over considerable distances and at a very low dilution by males.

Other species – grasshoppers and crickets, for example – use sound as a means of bringing the two sexes together. They do this by rubbing the upper part of their long hind legs against a ridge on their wing covers, or in crickets, by rubbing one wing cover against the other. Of course many insect sounds are involuntary, being caused by their wing beats.

Honey bees communicate with each other by performing little dances in the hive. This tells the onlookers that a source of food has been found, *where* it is, and how far from the hive – a truly remarkable piece of communication.

Far from advising how to get rid of wasps and bees, we should like to emphasize that they are valuable assets to the gardener as well as being interesting to watch. Wasps help to keep pest species under control, and bees pollinate our fruit and vegetables.

Of course both can sting, but only if disturbed. Wasps may attack if you stand too near the nest or if you gesticulate wildly when it comes near. Left alone it will go away.

Bees, however, have a barbed sting which usually remains in the flesh. This means it is torn out of the bee's body, and it dies – thus it will not sting unless there is good reason.

Honey bees are not, of course, native to Britain. They originate from Asia and so hibernate in the winter to which their ancestors weren't accustomed. In summer they increase by swarming – a queen with many thousands of bees will leave the hive and set up house elsewhere. Though it is terrifying to be near, they rarely sting at this time for they are far too busy. Having left the hive, they alight on a nearby branch or some other protrusion in a seething mass weighing several pounds, while scouts are sent out to find a new home. This is not an easy task for a forest-dwelling tropical insect, and needs the help of a friendly, human beekeeper. To keep the swarm from moving until he arrives it is useful to simulate rain (without drenching them) and thunder (by banging saucepans, etc.).

A great many insects are active at night and the most obvious are the moths. In fact, most of Britain's 2,000 or so species are nocturnal. However, they do need small amounts of light to become active and perhaps this explains why moths are so attracted, apparently compulsorily so, to artificial light.

Some species, the glow worm and fireflies, make their own light and in foreign countries (for we have only two species in Britain) they make dazzling displays. I have spent a fascinating evening by a hippo pool watching a dazzling display of fireflies. The light from these tiny creatures pulsating on and off as they wheeled to and fro. The light is produced by a chemical reaction which takes place when oxygen is directed to a substance called Luciferin in the presence of an enzyme. Even more extraordinary, in the case of the glow worm, is that at the back of this chemical is a layer of reflecting crystals which acts like a mirror to reflect all the light that is produced towards the outside. Apparently all the energy is converted into light with no wastage as heat; a lesson which men should learn in these days of energy crisis.

Not content with sharing the wild areas with us, insects invade our gardens and houses. Perhaps the most common and best known insect that invades our houses is the house fly (*musca domestica*). The common house fly, however, is actually far less common than it was 50 years ago, partly because of the widespread use of insecticide and also because of improved sanitation and a decline in the use of the horse – for the house fly breeds in dung and filth. For this reason and also the fact that it regurgitates fluid onto whatever food it wants to ingest, it is a dangerous carrier of germs.

Not so the common black cockroach which is a confirmed scavenger, and is found wherever there is food material in plentiful supply. It probably does a useful job in clearing up food debris and it certainly presents no threat to human beings, and its presence does *not* denote a dirty house. Perhaps it is so feared and hated because it is nocturnal; when you've got up to get a drink of water it *can* be a little spine chilling to see cockroaches scurrying away in the middle of the night. I must have done this once in Teheran – more than half asleep – for, when I came down to the kitchen the next morning I found my footsteps across the kitchen floor to the sink outlined in dead cockroaches!

Another house dweller, or perhaps one should say kitchen or pantry dweller, is the little silver fish which can be seen during the day as well as at night. It is a scavenger of food material as well as dead insects. They do us no harm, and perhaps a service in clearing up food particles.

Another insect about which most of us will have heard creepy stories in our youth is the earwig. The cause of the unpopularity, of course, is the generally accepted belief that they will crawl into your ears during the night. Though this is possible there have been very few reported cases, and certainly it would do absolutely no damage in the ear. More than likely it would turn round and come out again straight away. They, like the cockroach and silver fish, are scavengers and help tidy up the small food particles that the housewife does not see. It may interest the housewife to know that the female earwig is a very good mother, looking after her eggs until they hatch, and then the young, licking them when they hatch, and feeding them for a week or two.

The furniture beetle or woodworm, although common out of doors, is often seen in the house. Its natural habitat is dead wood and it finds tree stumps or sheds just as attractive as floorboards or furniture.

Ants prefer to live outside, but who can blame them if they make their nest indoors when there is a plentiful food supply? They are clean creatures that scavenge food particles and cause no harm to human beings unless handled roughly, of course, when they will sting. In the garden where they more commonly make their nest, they help to aerate the soil and kill quite a number of species of pests that damage garden plants. They also 'farm' and 'milk' aphids. They collect aphids and take them into their nests alive where they 'feed' them and, perhaps more commonly, they install the aphids in 'cow sheds' around the stems of plants. The aphids suck the juices from the plant and excrete a sweet fluid which the ants then consume. Ants sometimes even collect aphid eggs and store them during the winter. When they hatch in the spring, the ants carry the young aphids out to the plants for 'farming'. How the ants 'know' that the aphid eggs will hatch in the spring and produce the aphids which they want to 'farm' is explained by genetics, but how it arose in the first place is unknown.

Perhaps the most disliked and feared of all this group found in the house is the spider, in spite of the fact that all British species – of which there are 600 – are harmless to man. All spiders are carnivorous. Many make intricate webs of silk to catch their prey which they then subdue with a bite from their poisonous fangs. Some are jumping spiders that stalk their prey, whilst others simply run down their prey. All are much more common outside than in.

There are many insects that live closely to man in his garden, where many are disliked, and most are pests. But there is no doubt that the finishing touch to a beautiful flower garden is the sight of a butterfly making its erratic journeys from plant to plant. Alas, with the advent of modern pesticides they are not so common. A few may cause damage, like the large white to cabbage plants, but most are attracted to buddleia, stinging nettles and wild flowers and cause no damage to vegetables or fruit. To encourage them a corner of the garden should be allowed to become wild with nettles, brambles, dandelions and other wild plants for food for the caterpillars. In addition flowers that are attractive to butterflies can be cultivated; buddleia is the favourite, but lavender, ageratum, honesty, alyssum, petunia, nicotinia and michaelmas daisies all provide the adult with nectar.

In comparison to the fifteen or twenty species of butterflies seen commonly in British gardens, there are more than 2,000 species of moths. The wings of butterflies and most moths are covered with minute scales which give the colour and design, and it is these that rub off on the fingers when the wings are touched. The difference between butterflies and moths, apart from the former being active in daytime and the latter nocturnal, is that the antennae of butterflies end in small knobs. Most moths are garden pests in that they can do a considerable amount of damage to fruit and vegetables.

One can often hear people say 'what use is this or that', and it is usually dangerous insects, garden pests, or just plain nuisances that they are referring to. The insect most often spoken about in these terms is the wasp, for its sting is quite painful. But it is very protective of its young, and if anyone dares stand in front of the nest they are inviting trouble. However, as mentioned previously, it does far more good than harm in the garden as it preys upon many insects that gardeners look upon as pests, such as caterpillars.

Aphids, on the other hand, have little to commend them. They are direct competitors to man and spoil much more garden produce than they consume.

Similarly slugs and snails also attack and destroy large amounts of plants that the gardener has been carefully growing. Their only benefit seems to be as food for birds. But slugs and snails prefer rotting material and the untidy gardener, therefore, will have less to grumble about.

Worms, on the other hand, are very valuable to the gardener. Upwards of one million per acre may be found in good grasslands, but the numbers in gardens are much lower, due probably to repeated cultivation. Worms come to the surface in the evening, generally warm summer evenings, but rarely leave their burrows completely. They keep their tail end tucked into the burrow to facilitate a quick retreat while they search around for food or for each other for mating. But if you want to see them in the evening in your garden lawn, walk carefully, for worms are highly sensitive to vibration and a heavy footstep will send them immediately back into their burrows. Worms pass a tremendous amount of soil through their bodies which helps to break it down into fine material, and their burrows aerate the soil and allow drainage. They also drag dead leaves into the burrows which slowly rot away and enrich the soil. Worm casts on a lawn is a sign of a healthy soil. Some gardeners kill them because they find the worm casts unsightly, but all that is needed is a stiff brush to sweep them away. Better to have a healthy lawn and brush away the worm casts, than risk poor drainage and the invasion of coarse grasses and weeds.

Another useful garden insect is the delightful looking little ladybird which, in fact, is a voracious predator that consumes large quantities of aphids. They are also survivors, as the warning red colour indicates, for they taste unpleasant and are not eaten by birds. 'Look after the ladybird' should be the motto of all gardeners.

Cuckoo spit is not uncommon in our herbaceous borders. Inside this froth is a little nymph which has exuded the fluid and blown air into it to protect itself from desiccation until the adult frog-hopper – for that is what it is – emerges in late autumn. These little insects do look a bit like frogs, and they hop from one plant to another, laying their eggs in the autumn.

But perhaps the most startlingly attractive insect is the dragon-fly and not all gardens are fortunate enough to have them. They are also confirmed predators both as nymphs and adults, and can catch their prey in flight. Their flight is astounding to watch, as they move swiftly, turn, hover and can even fly backwards. They are only found near water.

Our enjoyment of the great outdoors is decreased to a certain extent by three main groups of insects: the mosquitoes, midges and hymenoptera (wasps, bees, ants, etc.). The hymenoptera are generally only bothersome when disturbed, but the mosquitoes and some species of midges are predators on man in that they are blood suckers. Female mosquitoes need a feed of blood before they can lay their eggs, while the male mosquitoes are content to feed on nectar and fruit juices and don't possess the piercing tube found in females. Both larvae and pupae develop in water, and mosquitoes and particularly midges are found most commonly in the moister parts of the British Isles. Fortunately, none of them carry any disease in Britain, but in tropical countries they do and one of the best ways to eradicate malaria would be to eradicate the mosquitoes that carry it.

Many readers will remember the timely warning given by Rachael Carson in her revolutionary book called *Silent Spring*, in which she highlighted the extensive use of pesticides, and showed how dangerous they were, by extension, to our bird life. Until the last war the pesticides used in agriculture and horticulture were harmless to birds and mammals. Pyrethrum is a naturally occurring product that was fairly effective in the control of many pests, and tar was used to spray on dormant fruit trees to protect them. Only derris was toxic and then only to fish, not to mammals or birds. Then synthetic poisons were discovered and one of the first was the most effective ever, known by the initials DDT. It is what is called an organo-chlorine compound and was produced in such vast quantities that traces of it can be found in the Arctic and Antarctic and in almost all forms of life. It was probably one of the most effective insecticides ever produced, but it had one important drawback: it was very persistent. Far from being biodegradable, it was taken up and concentrated at each trophic level (in the food chain). This meant that the top predators were consuming, in the bodies of their prey, relatively large amounts of DDT. At first it was thought to be non-poisonous to mammals and birds, but then it was discovered that when a sufficiently high level in the body was reached animals showed nervous symptoms, emaciation and diarrhoea. Birds, with a lower level of pesticide in their bodies, developed soft-shelled eggs and low fertility. All of the organo-chlorine compounds – Aldrin, Dialdrin and DDT as well as BHC – are persistent pesticides, and where possible should be avoided in the interests of ecology.

Following this, the organo-phosphorus compounds were discovered which, though just as dangerous, were not quite so persistent in the environment. Mevinphos was one of the first though other less persistent compounds are on the market. Needless to say all these compounds are highly toxic to man and protective clothing has to be worn when they are being used.

So if your garden is full of pests that you must get rid of and you do not want to contaminate the environment and endanger birds and mammals, what are you to do? Apart from using safe pesticides, such as pyrethrum or derris or tar oil, there are several ways of preventing infestation with pests before the trouble begins.

Carrot fly can be largely prevented by firming up the soil when the young carrots are at an early stage of growth, and planting shallots or chives between the rows. White fly and aphids are susceptible to nettle manure which is made by putting a bunch of nettles in a bucket of water and leaving them there for four days and then spraying the fluid onto and around the plants that are being attacked.

Slugs can be killed with Methaldihide. This is sold in most garden shops as slug bait, but remember that it can poison hedgehogs, so some form of covering should be put over the material (large cinders put around the area can be a deterrent, or wood shavings or straw). Slugs are particularly fond of beer and many gardeners find it useful to sink a jam pot with some beer in it at soil level which the slugs will then seek out and drop into. Another method is to put a leaf of rhubarb on the ground between your plants under which the slugs will seek shelter during the night. Early in the morning you simply pick up the leaves and throw them on the compost heap with the slugs attached to the underside.

Derris and pyrethrum are effective against caterpillars, and will not poison birds who are just as useful in reducing their numbers. The smell of lavender and thyme repels aphids.

Earwig

Common cockroach (black)

Death's head hawk moth

Dragon-fly

Ladybird

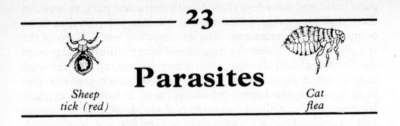

23

Parasites

*Sheep
tick (red)*

*Cat
flea*

The word itself makes one uneasy, but it is worth acknowledging that very few wild creatures are free of parasites, whether internal or external. In this chapter we will only glance briefly at their strange world.

Two childhood memories still make me shudder. One was when I picked up a baby swift that had fallen from the nest. It was alive, but unconscious and as I cradled it in my hand two huge (or so they seemed) flattened, crab-like insects scuttled rapidly onto my hand and up my arm. I shook them off in terror. The other was finding, on post mortem, that the intestines of a newly killed chicken were full of large white worms. I can remember wondering how the bird had managed to survive and what it may have suffered.

Some insects are parasitic at only one stage of their development, whilst others never leave the host, and their harmfulness to the host is largely dependent on their numbers and the reaction of the host to the parasite: for the parasite to survive successfully its host has to remain reasonably healthy. However, if the infestation is a large one, disease symptoms and even death can result.

External or ectoparasites are generally less likely to cause problems, and birds, for instance, have developed dust bathing, preening and, in certain species, 'anting' to keep these parasites under control. But this equilibrium between host and parasite can be upset by a lowering of the resistance of the birds due to weather conditions, food supply and unusual stresses when the parasites can multiply excessively.

It is perhaps a comforting thought that countless thousands of parasites never achieve their full life cycle. Vast numbers of immature ticks, for example, wait, clinging to vegetation, in vain hope that a suitable host will brush past within reach.

Parasites that produce eggs, do so by the million to ensure survival; some species reproduce asexually and others do not and often experience great difficulty in finding a mate.

Many internal parasites absorb food through the surface of

their body and have lost their mouth parts and part, at least, of their digestive organs, and almost all internal parasites have complicated life cycles involving intermediate hosts. Many of the species of flukes infecting birds have seven different stages of development: first the egg, then a free swimming, tadpole-like stage, then a cystic stage within the host, then another free swimming stage and another cystic stage in an intermediate host which can be anything from mammals and amphibia to jellyfish and even leeches, and finally the mature parasite in the bird. Some species of tapeworm found in foxes use the flea as the intermediate host.

Most internal parasites are host specific or are restricted to hosts closely resembling each other.

Worms

There are four types of parasitic worms: round worms, tape worms and flukes, spiny headed and segmented worms (leeches). Only the last group contain some free living species. The other three are parasitic, produce millions of eggs with an intermediate stage in another host – for some tape worms it is the flea and for some flukes, snails or dragon-flies.

The round worms have a simple cycle within one host, and most species are found in the intestines but some attack other organs such as the lungs, kidneys and even the heart and the eyes. Many species hatch and develop outside the animal, but some go through the intermediate stage in the blood of their hosts. Post mortems have shown the blood of wild birds to be occasionally teeming with larval worms.

The spiny headed worms, which have hooks to attach themselves to the host, are mainly parasitic of fish, though a few are found in birds.

External or Ectoparasites

These are not so strongly host specific as the internal parasitic worms, except perhaps for lice. Though even with lice there is one interesting exception in that human lice will feed and breed on pigs, and the pig louse is equally at home on humans.

Ectoparasites are less likely to cause immune reactions, and while flea bites, for instance, can irritate, they may account for birds 'anting'. This is quite amusing to watch as the afflicted birds will squat and spread their wings on top of an ants' nest so that they become covered in the insects, others will pick up the ants and thrust them under the feathers. Often the abdomens of the ants are burst by the bird's beak, which probably releases the formic acid which may act as a repellent to fleas and lice.

The blood-sucking parasites have developed a type of saliva that prevents blood from clotting and have lost the sensory organs of eyes and ears. These fleas and lice parasitize all vertebrates, and they are more of a nuisance to humans than a hazard except that some can carry disease. They have a hard, resistant shell, and claws adapted for clinging. Fleas are flattened from side to side and lice from above to below. Fleas have a metamorphosis, i.e. pupa formation in their development, which takes place away from the host. Lice on the other hand merely moult to grow. On mammals these parasites live on blood, but on birds the feather louse chews on feathers for food.

Flat flies or louse flies are a highly specialized species. They are large – $\frac{1}{4}$in. long. To the swift they would be as large as a sizeable crab to humans, and as many as 20 have been found on a single bird. They are bloodsuckers, have wings, which in some species are vestigial, and seem to 'fly' sideways in a hopping manner which most people find rather revolting. They do bite, but this is neither dangerous nor painful. And they produce only one egg at a time which is hatched inside the insect and is born as a larvae which immediately pupates for the whole winter and hatches in the spring.

Mosquitoes, blackflies and midges are common parasitic bloodsuckers which mainly attack mammals, though a few species are specific to birds. They are notorious disease carriers, for example wild duck are susceptible to a malaria type parasite which is carried by blackflies, and the blackfly can also carry a group of worms called onchocerca.

A parasite which can kill its host is the green bottle, which is attracted to wounds on which it lays its numerous eggs. The larva, when hatched, then begin to devour the host.

Mites are very small – almost microscopic, spider-shaped creatures that either live on the skin or burrow into it causing the disease we call mange in mammals. Red mites are larger and are found in the nests of birds whose blood they suck from time to time.

Feather mites are not bloodsuckers, but feed on skin cells and feathers as their name suggests.

The lung mite can also affect birds attacking the bronchial tubes and air sacs.

Ticks are also a species of mite, and they are found on both mammals and birds. They are unpleasant parasites for their saliva is toxic and one bite can sometimes kill a bird, and cause illness in mammals. Even the eggs contain poisonous substances, and, in common with most biting, bloodsucking insects, ticks can transmit diseases.

APPENDICES

Appendix A
Wildlife and the Law

Official protection of wildlife from destruction and cruelty began comparatively recently. One of the earliest legal steps taken was the Sea Bird Protection Act of 1869, and then in 1872 the Wild Birds Protection Act was passed which covered seventy-nine species. Other acts followed but not until 1904 was an act passed to reduce cruelty by banning the pole trap. Several acts followed banning the teagle (a baited tene for catching birds) and birdlime.

In 1911 the Protection of Animals Act was passed in England and Wales, and a similar act in Scotland in 1912, and they are still in force. These acts give protection to domestic and captive animals but not to free living wild creatures. They prohibit the infliction of suffering both physical and mental and define the parameters. It is an offence, for instance, to cause suffering by omitting to do certain necessary things such as feeding and watering, and milking a cow. Certain practices are excluded such as hunting, coursing and slaughtering. But when a wild creature is confined for the purpose of treatment and nursing it too enjoys the protection of this Act. It must not be treated cruelly or starved unnecessarily, nor must it be released in an injured or crippled state unable to fend for itself.

The Grey Seals Protection Act passed in 1932 was replaced in 1970 by the Conservation of Seals Act. Its main purpose was to control the methods of killing and prohibit the use of poisons, and it gave powers to the Secretary of State to license killing.

Under the Destructive Imported Animals Act 1932 (Grey Squirrels Order 1937) it may be considered an offence to keep and/or release a grey squirrel except under licence.

Bird protection legislation was updated in 1954 and amended in 1967 and 1976 to give added cover. Now all wild birds, their nests and eggs, are protected by law with only a few exceptions, these being 'pest' species and sporting birds, and for certain purposes such as treatment of the sick and injured. There are four schedules in the Act. The first contains a list of birds that are specially protected at all times, and a small list of birds that are protected during the close season, February 1 to August 31. The second contains birds which may be killed or taken by authorized persons. The third list are birds which may be taken *outside* the close season – usually the same dates as above. And the fourth schedule contains those that may not be sold alive unless bred in captivity and close-ringed (a term describing a ring put on a fledgling and irremovable).

You may capture any sick or injured bird and kill it to relieve suffering, or treat it, provided it is properly cared for whilst in captivity and released once it has fully recovered.

The Pests Act of 1954 is concerned with regulating the methods used to control pests. Only certain types of traps are allowed and the spreading of myxomatosis is prohibited.

The Game Laws are designed to protect certain game from being hunted to extinction, and so they establish close seasons when game may not be taken. The Deer Act of 1963 is undergoing amendment as this book is being written. As it stands it establishes close seasons and times, and makes some weapons and ammunition unlawful. One important exception is, of course, when an animal is suffering from injury or disease.

The Badgers Act of 1974 protects this animal not only from being killed or taken but from being cruelly treated. Again taking for treatment, and killing when treatment is considered impossible, are excepted. So too is the taking and killing to protect agriculture.

The Protection of Animals (Anaesthetics) Acts of 1954 and 1964 require that for operations involving sensitive tissues and bone, which cause pain, a suitable anaesthetic must be used. Birds were exempted in the 1954 Act, but for a major operation an anaesthetic should be used.

The Veterinary Surgeons Act of 1966, which does include birds, restricts the practice of veterinary surgery to registered veterinary surgeons and practitioners, and defines the practice as the diagnosis of disease, giving advice based on that diagnosis, medicinal and surgical treatment, and the performance of operations. However, with the exception of operations requiring an anaesthetic and the use of scheduled drugs, first-aid treatment to any wild animal is exempted; and any treatment given by an owner of an animal or member of the owner's household or an employee is also exempted if such treatment is applied to the owned animal. If in any doubt as to your rights, consult your local RSPCA Inspector.

The Transit of Animals (General) Order of 1973 requires that animals must not be transported in a manner likely to cause suffering.

The Dangerous Wild Animals Act of 1976 was passed to

protect the public and applies to dangerous animals listed in the schedule and requires prospective owners to obtain a licence before being allowed to keep them.

Finally, in 1975 the Conservation of Wild Creatures and Wild Plants Act was passed to protect those endangered species on the schedule. Six animals and twenty-one plants were listed when the Act was passed. Since then the large blue butterfly has been declared extinct, and the otter in England and Wales was added to the schedule in January 1978. Other animals included are the greater horse-shoe bat, the mouse-eared bat, the sand lizard, the smooth snake and the natterjack toad. It is an offence to kill, injure, take (or attempt to do so), or to have in one's possession any creatures on the schedule. As before, it is allowed to take a listed creature that is disabled in order to tend it or to kill it if it is so seriously injured or in such a condition that to do so would be an act of mercy.

Since its inception, the Council of Europe has been considering, among other things, the conservation and protection of animals. Already there has been a directive on bird conservation which not only protects certain species from being killed, but also prohibits certain methods of taking those birds which are not listed. There have also been directives on the conservation of migratory species of wild animals, and on the protection of habitats. Once agreed by the Ministers, the participating countries are obliged to pass legislation within their countries to conform to the directives. At the present time a bill called 'The Wild Creatures and Plant Bill' is being prepared in Britain to conform to this directive.

These then are the main laws relating to caring for wildlife. There are other laws which may occasionally apply. The civil law has not been mentioned for it has many ramifications, and the advice of a solicitor should be sought if there is any chance of liability.

Appendix B
Euthanasia

From the purely technical point of view it is most difficult to describe methods of humanely killing birds and small mammals. A humane death, from the animal's point of view, is instantaneous without any excessive previous stress – such as blowing its head off with a gun while it is quietly resting. However, because the person called upon to kill is usually sensitive, kind, and reluctant to do so except to relieve suffering, the method must be acceptable and fairly easy to do without any special equipment. The simplest course of action is to take the unfortunate creature to the expert – a veterinary surgeon or an RSPCA Inspector. This is not always possible, and so we describe below methods which are *practical*, but in no way can we claim that they are anything but unpleasant.

Small birds and mammals can be killed by crushing their heads quickly with a stone or your heel, or you can hold them in one hand and swing them sharply down so that the back of the neck and head strikes the edge of a hard ledge. Larger birds can be killed by dislocating the neck. However this does require a fair amount of strength if the neck is pulled. Alternatively, it can be dislocated or broken with a sharp blow of a stick just behind the head with the bird held so that the head is hanging down. A method for a goose or swan is to lay its head on the ground, put a stick across the neck, stand on it and pull the body sharply upwards. This is best carried out after the bird has been stunned with a sharp blow to the head with a stick.

An overdose of the anaesthetic, ether, may be used. However, it is highly inflammable, and not easily obtained. To put a blackbird to sleep, for example, put 2 teaspoonfuls on a wad of cotton wool, and place it beside the bird in a small box just big enough to hold it. The box should be completely airtight until the animal is unconscious, and the operation will take about 5–10 minutes.

The neck of a rabbit is dislocated with a sharp blow with the edge of one hand or a heavy short stick, while the animal is held with its head dangling down.

Larger animals should be shot. A 12-bore shotgun at point-blank range will kill any animal smaller than a deer if placed just above the eyes and pointing down the spine (perpendicular to the skull). The assistance of an experienced marksman should be sought for deer. Use of guns is, of course, restricted to those with a licence to own and use them.

Symptoms of death are: absence of respiration and heartbeat, and failure to respond to painful stimuli.

To kill fish, just stun with a blow to the head and if strong enough it will kill. It is best to use a loaded or weighted club called a priest, that is purpose made, and sold by fishing-tackle merchants. The blow should be applied to the top of the skull just in front of where the ear might be – but not *too* far forward.

Very small fish can be killed by throwing them hard on the ground. Flat fish are harder to kill and eels are best killed by severing the head from the body after being stunned with a blow from the priest.

Close Seasons: Mammals

	Jan	Feb	Mar	Apr	May	June	July	Aug	Sept	Oct	Nov	Dec
Deer												
Fallow:												
Buck				1st		31st						
Doe		1st							31st			
Red:												
Stag				1st		31st						
Hind	1st								31st			
Roe:												
Doe	1st								31st			
Sika:												
Stag				1st		31st						
Hind	1st								31st			
Seal												
Common					1st		31st					
Grey									1st			31st

Close Seasons
Open Seasons

Note: There is no close season for hares, but they may not be killed on Sundays or on Christmas Day. On moorland or non-arable land, only the legal occupier may kill hares.

Appendix C
Close Seasons: Birds

	Jan	Feb	Mar	Apr	May	June	July	Aug	Sept	Oct	Nov	Dec
Capercaillie		1st							30th			
Coot		1st						31st				
Curlew		1st						31st				
Duck		1st						31st				
Geese		1st						31st				
Grouse								11th				11th
Moorhen		1st						31st				
Partridge		2nd						31st				
Pheasant		2nd								2nd		
Plover (Golden & Grey)		1st						31st				
Redshank (common)		1st						31st				
Snipe		1st						11th				
Whimbrel		1st						31st				
Woodcock		1st							30th			

Close Seasons
Open Seasons

Appendix D

Organizations

Bird Hospital Society, 58 Aldbourne Road, London W12. 01 749 4373

British Deer Society, Stede Court, Ashford, Kent. Ashford 291235.

British Trust for Ornithology, Beech Grove, Tring, Hertfordshire. Tring 3461.

County Naturalists' Trusts, Refer to local telephone directory.

Fauna and Flora Preservation Society, c/o Zoological Society of London, Regents Park, London, NW1 4RY. 01 586 0872.

The Mammal Society, Harvest House, Reading, RG1. Reading 861345.

Nature Conservancy Regional Officers, Refer to local telephone directory.

The Otter Trust, Earsham, nr. Bungay, Suffolk. Bungay 3470.

People's Trust for Endangered Species, 19 Quarry Street, Guildford, Surrey. Guildford 35671.

RSPCA Headquarters (Wildlife Department), The Manor House, The Causeway, Horsham, Surrey. Horsham 64181.

RSPCA Local Inspector, Refer to local telephone directory.

RSPCA Wildlife Field Unit, Little Creech, West Hatch, Taunton, Somerset. Hatch Beauchamp 480156.

RSPB Headquarters, The Lodge, Sandy, Bedfordshire. Sandy 80551.

RSPB Regional officers and reserves, Refer to local telephone directory.

Aberdeen SPCA, 6 Bon Accord Square, Aberdeen, AB9 1XU. Aberdeen 21 236.

Glasgow & West of Scotland SPCA, 15 Royal Terrace, Glasgow, G3 7NY. Glasgow 332 0716.

Scottish SPCA, 19 Melville Street, Edinburgh, E3 7PL. Edinburgh 225 6418.

Royal Society for Nature Conservation, The Green, Nettleham, Lincoln. Lincoln 52326.

Wildfowl Trust, Slimbridge, Gloucestershire, GL2 7BT. Cambridge (Glos.) 333.

The Wildfowl Trust, Mill Road, Arundel, West Sussex. Arundel 883355.

The Wildfowl Trust, Martin Nere, Burscough, Ormskirk, Lancashire. Burscough 895181.

The Wildfowl Trust, Middle Barnston Farn, Washington 15, Tyne and Wear. Washington 465456.

The Wildfowl Trust, Peakirk, Peterborough, Cambridgeshire. Peakirk 252271.

The Wildfowl Trust, Pintail House, Hundred Foot Bank, Welney, Wisbech. Welney 860711.

The Wildfowl Trust, East Park Farn, Caeroaverock, Dumfriesshire. Caeroaverock 200.

Appendix E

Wild Animals of Britain

The following lists, particularly in the bird chapters, are selected specifically for this book. They are not intended to conform to any particular scientific pattern. The blackbird and the robin, for instance, are also members of the thrush family but are listed separately since they are more likely to be encountered as casualties than some of the other family members.

Birds

Chapter 1
Swans (three species)
Geese (eight species)
Ducks (eighteen species)

Chapter 2
Grebes (four species)
Divers (three species)
Gulls (six species)
Terns (five species)
Guillemots (two species)
Skuas (two species)
Gannet
Manx Shearwater
Cormorant
Shag
Fulmar
Razorbill
Puffin
Petrels (two species)

Chapter 3
Corncrake
Curlews (two species)
Greenshank
Plovers (four species)
Lapwing
Dotterel

Woodcock
Bittern
Heron
Water Rail
Spotted Crake
Snipe (two species)
Godwit (two species)
Ruff
Phalaropes (two species)
Sandpipers (five species)
Redshank
Greenshank
Dipper
Moorhen
Coot
Spoonbill
Avocet
Whimbrel
Dunlin
Knot
Sanderling
Turnstone
Oystercatcher

Chapter 4
Pheasant
Partridges (two species)

Quail
Grouse (two species)
Ptarmigan
Capercaillie

Chapter 5
Owls (five species)
Kestrel
Harriers (three species)
Hobby
Merlin
Golden Eagle
Sparrowhawk
Red Kite
Buzzards (three species)
Osprey
Peregrine
Goshawk

Chapter 6
Starling
Sparrows (three species)
Martins (two species)
Thrushes (ten species)
Robin
Tits (eight species)

Swift
Doves (four species)
Blackbird
Wren
Finches (sixteen species)
 (inc. Buntings)
Waxwing
Wood-pigeon
Swallow
Nightjar
Shrikes (four species)
Pipits (three species)
Treecreeper
Goldcrest
Kingfisher
Flycatchers (two species)
Hoopoe
Crows (eight species)
Larks (three species)
Cuckoo
Warblers (twelve species)
Woodpeckers (four
 species)
Nuthatch
Firecrest
Wagtails (three species)

Mammals

Chapter 8
Mole
Dormice (two species)
Mice (four species)
Shrews (three species)
Voles (three species)
Rats (two species)

Chapter 9
Bats (fifteen species)

Chapter 10
Hedgehog

Chapter 11
Rabbit
Hares (two species)

Chapter 12
Squirrels (two species)

Chapter 13
Pine Marten
Weasel
American Mink
Stoat
Polecat
Ferret

Chapter 14
Fox

Chapter 15
Otter

Chapter 16
Seals (two species)
Whales (at least fifteen
 species stranded on
 U.K. coasts)

Dolphins (at least
seven species
stranded on U.K.
coasts)

Chapter 17
Badger

Chapter 18
Deer (six species)

Chapter 19
Snakes (three species)
Lizards (three species)

Chapter 20
Frogs (three species –
two imported and
very rare)
Toads (two species)
Newts (three species)

Index

Page numbers in italics refer to illustrations

Adder, 156, *156*, 157, 159
Aldrin, 175
Alpha-Chlorolose, 27
American mink, 115
Amphibia, 160–2
 capture, 161
 food, 162
 handling hazards, 161
 initial care, 101
 release, 162
 symptoms, diagnosis and
  treatment, 162
 transportation, 161
 See also under individual species
Ants, 171, 172, 177
Aphids, 171, 173, 175
 cabbage, 168
Arabian Sea, 167
Ashby, Eric, 116
Aspergillosis, 27, 73
Auk, 28, 70, 71, 72, 76, 77
Avian tuberculosis, 41

Badger, 132, 138–146, *142*
 approach and capture, 139–40
 food, 141
 force-feeding, 141
 general care, 144
 initial care, 141
 orphans, 145–6
 possible handling hazards, 139
 release, 144–5
 symptoms, diagnosis and
  treatment, 142–4
 transportation, 141
Badgers Act 1974, 181
Bank vole, 82
Barn owl, *53*

Bat, 87–90
 approach and capture, 88
 food, 89
 general care, 89–90
 great or noctule, 87, *90*
 greater horseshoe, *87*, 88, 182
 initial care, 89
 long-eared, 87, *89*
 mouse-eared, 88, 182
 natterer's, 87
 pipistrelle, 87, *89*
 possible handling hazards, 88
 symptoms, diagnosis and
  treatment, 89
 transportation, 89
 whiskered, 87
Bed bugs, 169
Bees, 169
 honey, 169, 170
BHC, 175
Birds of prey (or raptors), 45–53
 approach and capture, 46–7
 food, 48–9
 force-feeding, 49
 general care, 50–1
 initial care, 47–8
 orphans, 52–3
 possible handling hazards, 46
 release, 51–2
 symptoms, diagnosis and
  treatment, 50
 transportation, 47
Bittern, 31
Blackbird, 65, *65*
 euthanasia of, 183
Blackflies, 178
Black rat, 81, 82–3
Blue tit, *62*

Blue whale, 163
Botulism, 17, 27
Bristol Zoo, 116
British Deer Society, 154
British grass snake, 157, *157*, 158, 159
Brown (or common) rat, 80, *80*, 81
Brucellosis, 85
Budgies, 64
Bumblefoot, 18
Butterfly, 172
  large blue, 182
  large white, 172
Buzzard, 49, *49*, 50

Cancers, 151
Capercaillie, 38
Carrot fly, 175
Carson, Rachel (*Silent Spring*), 174
Chaffinch, 67
Chinese water deer, 147, 153, *153*
Close seasons, birds, 185
  mammals, 186
Cockroach, 170, 171
  common (black), 170, *171*
Cod, 164
Conservation of Seals Act 1970, 180
Common toad, 160
Complan, 136
Conservation of Wild Creatures and Wild Plants Act 1975, 182
Coot, 31, *31*, 36
Council of Europe, 182
County Naturalist's Trust, 126, 145, 154
Cranbrook, Lord, 165
Cricket, 169
Crow, 57, *57*, 58, 59, 64, 67, 68
Cruelty to Wild Animals, government committee on, 166
Cuckoo, 45

Dangerous Wild Animals Act 1976, 181-2
DDT, 174, 175

Deer, 146-54
  approach and capture, 148
  Chinese water, 147, 153, *153*
  euthanisia of, 184
  fallow, 146, *150*
  food, 149
  force-feeding, 149-50
  general care, 152
  initial care, 149
  muntjac, 146, *154*
  orphans, 152-4
  possible handling hazards, 148
  red, 146, *146*
  roe, 146, *151*, 153
  sika, 146, *149*
  symptoms, diagnosis and treatment, 150-2
  transportation, 148-9
  See also under individual species
Deer Act 1967, 181
Derris, 175
Destructive Imported Animals Act 1932 (Grey Squirrels Order Act 1937), 180
Dettol, 13
Diadrin, 175
Dichlorxylenol, 42
Diver, 28, 71, 72
Dolphin, 133, 134, 135
  bottle-nosed, 133
  common, 133
Dormouse, 80, 82, *82*, 84
  edible, 80
Dragon-fly, 173-4, *174*
Duck, 6, 8, 10, 11
  food, 10
  force-feeding, 10-12
  mallard, male, *19*
  orphans, 19

Earwig, 171, *171*
Eel, 165
  freshwater, 165
  yellow, 165
Enkephalin, 166
Enteritis, 73
Entorphine (M99), 150
Euthanasia, 183-4

Falconry, 47
Fallow deer, 146, *150*
Ferret, 115
Fieldfare, 66
Finch, 57, 67
  foreign, 64
Fireflies, 170
Fish, 163–7
  euthanasia of, 184
  See also under individual species
Flatflies, 178
Flea, 169, 177
  cat, *178*
Flycatcher, pied, *60*
Foot and mouth disease, 151
Fox, 116–127, *121*
  approach, capture and
    transportation, 117–18
  cub, *126*
  food, 119
  general care, 122–4
  initial care, 118–19
  orphans, 125–7
  outdoor pen for, *123*
  possible handling hazards, 117
  symptoms, diagnosis and
    treatment, 119–20
Frog-hopper, 173
Frog, 160–1
  common or grass, 161, *161*
Fulmar, 29

Game (?) birds, 38–44
  food, 40
  force-feeding, 40
  general care, 42
  initial care, 40
  orphans, 43–4
  possible handling hazards, 39
  release, 43
  symptoms, diagnosis and
    treatment, 40–1
  transportation, 39
  See also under individual species
Game Laws, 181
Gannet, 22, *25*, 71, *72*
Gape worm, 42
Gapex, 42

Geese, 6, 7, 8, 10
  euthanasia of, 183
  orphans, 19
Glow worm, 170
Goldcrest, 56, 63, *64*
Goose, *see* Geese
Grasshopper, 169
  common, *169*
Grasshopper warbler, 66
Grass snake, 157, *157*, 158, 159
Great tit, *59*
Grebe, 23, 71
Green bottle, 178
Grey squirrel, 105, *106*
Grey Seals Protection Act 1939,
  180
Grouse, red, 42
Guillemot, *25*, 70, 71
Gulf Stream, 165
Gull, 23, 25, 28

Hare, 99–104
  blue, 99
  brown, 99, *100*
Harvest mouse, 84, *84*, 85
Hedgehog, 91–8, *94*, 175
  approach and capture, 92
  food, 93–4
  force-feeding, 94
  general care, 95
  initial care, 92–3
  orphans, 96–8
  possible handling hazards,
    92
  release, 95–6
  symptoms, diagnosis and
    treatment, 94–5
  transportation, 92
Hen or bantam, broody, 19, 43
Heron, 31, 34, 35, *35*, 36, 37
Herring, 164
Herring gull, 25, *27*, 28
Hoopoe, 56
Horse flies, 169
House fly (*musca domestica*),
  170
House mouse, 81
Hymenoptera, 176

Infectious anaemia, 85
Insects, 168–75
  See also under individual species

Kaobotic, 73
Kestrel, 49, *49*, 50
  foot of, *45*
Kingfisher, 56, *56*, 60

Lactol, 126, 131, 150, 153
Ladybird, 173, *173*
Lead poisoning, 15, 16
Leech, 177
Leptospirosis, 85, 95, 108, 131
Lice, 169, 177, 178
  human, 177
  pig, 177
Little owl, *45*, 46, 50
Little tern, 22, *22*
Lizard, 156–9
  common, 157
  sand, 157, *157*, 182
Long-tailed fieldmouse (or wood
  mouse), 82, 84
Long-tailed tit, *69*
Louse flies, 178
Luciferin, 170
Lymenoptera, 174

Malathion, 121
Mallard duck, *19*, 71
  ducklings, 36
Mange, in foxes, 122
Manx shearwater, 29–30
Mebenvet, 42
Merlin, 45
Methaldihide, 175
Mevinphos, 175
Mice, *see* Mouse
Midges, 169, 174, 178
Ministry of Agriculture,
  Fisheries and Food, 27, 143,
  144
Mink, American, 115
Mistle thrush, 57
Mites, 178
  feather, 178
  lung, 178

Mole, 80, *80*, 82, 84, 85
Moorhen, 31, 36
Mosquito, 169, 174, *174*, 178
Moth, 169, 170, 172
  death's head hawk, 168, *170*
Mouse, 80–86
  harvest, 84, *84*, 85
  house, 81
  long-tailed field, 81, 84
Muntjac deer, 146, *154*
Mute swan, 6, 71
Myco-bacterial diseases, 41
Myxomatosis, 102

Natterjack toad, 160, 161, *161*
Newt, 160, 161
  common, male, *161*
  crested, male, *161*
  palmate, male, *161*
Nine-spined stickleback, *163*

Oil pollution, 70–77
Onchocerca, 178
Organizations, 187
Otter Trust, The, 131
Otter, 71, 128–32, *129*, 182
  approach and capture, 129–30
  food, 130
  general care, 131
  initial care, 130
  orphans, 131–2
  possible handling hazards, 129
  release, 131
  symptoms, diagnosis and
    treatment, 130–1
Owl, 45, 46, 47, 50, 52, 53
  barn, *53*
  little, *45*, 46, 50
  tawny, 45, 46, 50, 52
Oxytetracyclin, 74

Parakeet, 64
Parasites, 151, 176–8
  external (or ectoparasites), 176,
    177–8
  internal, 176–7
Parathion, 121
Partridge, male, *40*

Penguin, 74
Perrins, Dr., 71
Perruque head, 151
Pests Act 1954, 181
Pheasant, 38, 39, 40, 41, 42, 50, 65
    male, *39*
Pied flycatcher, 60
Pigmy shrew, 80, *81*
Pine marten, 111, 113, *113*, 114
Pipistrelle, 87, *89*
Plover (lapwing), *36*
    ringed, 31
Polecat, 111, *111*, 114
Porpoise, common, 133
Protection of Animals
    (Anaesthetics) Acts 1954 and
    1964, 181
Protection of Animals Act 1911,
    166
Protection of Animals Act
    (England and Wales) 1911,
    180 (Scotland) 1912, 180
Psittacosis, 41, 63
Puffin, 71, *71*
Pyrethrum, 175

Quail, 38, *42*

Rabbit, 99–104, *101*
    euthanasia of, 183
Raptors, *see* Birds of prey
Rat, 80–3
    black, 81, 82–3
    brown, 80, *80*
Raven, 56, 57, 65
Razorbill, 71, *71*
Red deer, 146, *146*
Red grouse, 42
Red squirrel, 105, *108*
Reptiles, *see* Snakes and lizards
Ringed plover, 31
Ring of Bright Water, 128
Robin, *58*
Roe deer, 146, *151*, 153
Royal Society for the Protection
    of Birds, 50
RSPCA, 137, 148, 152, 154,
    181, 183

Salmon, 163, 165
Salmonella, salmonellosis, 41,
    63, 85, 95
Sargasso Sea, 165
Sea Bird Protection Act 1869,
    180
Sea Duck, 71
Seal, 71, 133, 136
    common, 133, *134*
    grey, 133
Shark, 165
Sheep-tick (red), *176*
Shrew, 80, 81, 84, 85
    common, 82
    water, 82, 86
    pigmy, *81*
Silent Death, 50
Silver fish, 171
Slow worm, 157–8, *158*
Slug, 173, 175
Smooth snake, 157, *157*, 182
Snail, 173
Snakes and lizards, 156–9
    approach and capture, 158
    food, 159
    general care, 159
    initial care, 159
    possible handling hazards, 158
    release, 159
    symptoms, diagnosis and
        treatment, 159
    transportation, 158
    See also under individual species
Snake, British grass, 157, *157*,
    158, 159
    smooth, 157, *157*, 182
Society for the Promotion of
    Nature Conservation, 90
Song thrush, *61*
Sparrow, *61*
Sparrowhawk, 45
Spider, 172
    garden, *172*
Spoonbill, 31
Squirrel, 105–10
    approach and capture, 105–6
    food, 106–7
    force-feeding, 107

general care, 108–9
grey, 105, *106*
initial care, 106
orphans, 109–10
possible handling hazards, 105
red, 105, *108*
symptoms, diagnosis and
    treatment, 107–8
transportation, 106
release, 109
Stag beetle, 168, *168*
Staphyloccal infection,
    staphyloccus, 18, 27, 74
Starling, *63*
Stoat, 111, *113*, 114
Straits of Messina, 165
Strychnine, 85
Swallow, 65, *65*
Swan, 6, 7, 8, 9, 10, 11, 12, 71
    euthanasia of, 183
    mute, 6, 7, 8, 9, 71
Swift, 46, 56, 60, 65

Tarka the Otter, 128
Teal, 11
    force-feeding, 11–12
Tern, little, 22, *22*
Tetramisole, 42
Thrush,
    mistle, 57
    song, *61*
Tick, 178
Tit,
    blue, *62*
    great, *59*
    long-tailed, 69
Toad, 160–1
    common, 160
    natterjack, 160, 161, *161*
Transit of Animals (General)
    Order 1973, 181

Treecreeper, 59, *59*
Trichostrongylus tenuis, 42
Trout, *164*
Tuberculosis, 42, 63, 138, 143,
    151

Veterinary Surgeons Act 1966,
    181
Vole, 80, *82*, 86
    bank, 82
    water, 86

Warfarin, 85, 121
Wasp, *169*, 172–3
    ichneumon, 169
Weasel, 111, 114, 115, *115*
Whale, 133, 134
    blue, 163
    pilot, 133
    sperm, 133
White fly, 175
Wild Birds Protection Act 1872,
    180
Wild Creatures and Plants Bill,
    182
Woodpecker, 59
    green, *60*
Wood-pigeon, 57, *57*
Woodworm, or furniture beetle,
    171
Worms, 173, 177
    flukes, 177
    leeches, 177
    round, 177
    tape, 177

Yellow-necked mouse, 84

Zoology department of
    Newcastle University, 70

Care for the Wild

Care for the Wild is a British charity, formed to represent people who want wild animals to be protected from killing and cruelty and from having their life-giving habitat destroyed. It is the only British charity with this mandate.

This book is only a small part of what Care for the Wild supporters have accomplished. They have made it possible for effective animal protection programmes to be funded and developed in Australia, Sri Lanka, Brazil, Bolivia, North America, Kenya, Rawanda and here at home. Harp seals, grey seals, pilot whales, humpback whales, sea turtles, otters, barn owls, elephants, rhinoceros, jaguars, kangaroos and many, many other wild animals have all directly benefited from the dedication, support, and concerns of Care for the Wild people.

You can become a valuable part of the work being done to protect wild animals in Britain and around the world by supporting Care for the Wild. Write, sending your name, address and a small donation, to:

> Care for the Wild
> 26 North Street
> Dept. BK
> Horsham
> West Sussex
> RH12 1BN

You compassion and generosity are the only things that stand between the wild animals and the human greed, cruelty, and ignorance that has caused – and continues to cause – so much suffering and death in the animal world. Support the protection of wild animals; support Care for the Wild.